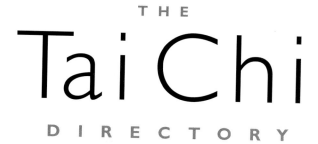

THE

Tai Chi

DIRECTORY

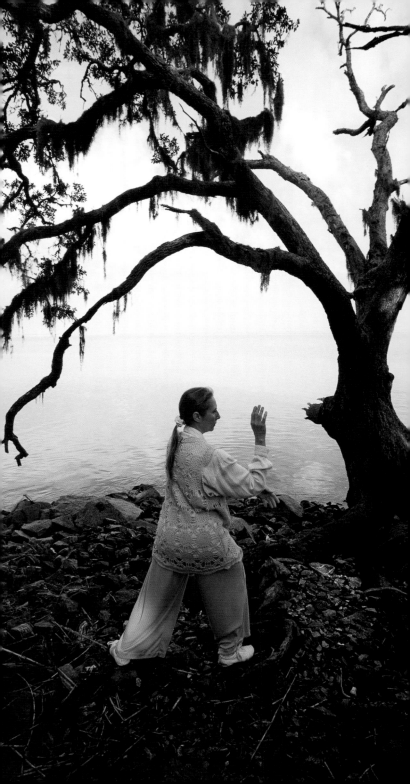

THE
Tai Chi
DIRECTORY

Kim Davies

METRO BOOKS
NEW YORK

Note from the publisher
This book should be considered as a reference source only and it
is not intended to replace instruction or advice from a qualified
practitioner or other healthcare professional. The author and
publisher disclaim any liability, loss, injury, or damage incurred
as a consequence, directly or indirectly, of the use and
application of the contents.

This book was conceived, designed, and produced by
Ivy Press
210 High Street, Lewes,
East Sussex, BN7 2NS, UK

CREATIVE DIRECTOR Peter Bridgewater
PUBLISHER Sophie Collins
EDITORIAL DIRECTOR Steve Luck
SENIOR PROJECT EDITOR Rebecca Saraceno
DESIGN MANAGER Tony Seddon
DESIGNER Kevin Knight
ARTWORK ASSISTANT Joanna Clinch
STUDIO PHOTOGRAPHY Guy Ryecart

Metro Books
122 Fifth Avenue
New York, NY 10011

ISBN: 978-1-4351-0881-3

Printed in China

3 5 7 9 10 8 6 4 2

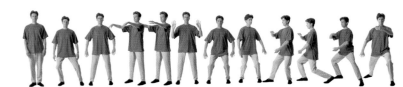

Contents

Introduction

As recently as thirty years ago, Eastern health systems were considered exotic curiosities. Most people viewed practices such as tai chi, yoga, and acupuncture with skepticism or disbelief—if they knew about them at all. And the medical profession looked askance at any medical or therapeutic wisdom that originated outside the Western clinical tradition.

But this has changed in the last generation or so. It is now widely accepted that Eastern philosophies are based on a deep understanding of the body. As a result, many of the ideas that underpin tai chi are now seen as complementary to Western understanding, rather than contradictory of it.

Scientific research has also validated many of the claims made for tai chi by its practitioners: studies have found, for example, that regular practice can reduce stress levels, and improve physical balance and muscular flexibility. Doctors now commonly recommend tai chi as a relaxation technique and as a form of physical exercise.

Tai chi in the West

The popularity of tai chi is one manifestation of a growing interest in—one might even call it a hunger for—the wisdom of Eastern cultures. In addition, the pioneering Westerners who learned from Chinese masters have had many years to refine their practice. There is now a generation of senior Western teachers, and they have helped to demystify tai chi and make it more accessible to people who have no special knowledge of the culture from which it emerged.

And the new students of this ancient practice finds that tai chi meets a real and urgent need. Stress and anxiety have become endemic problems in our fast-driven society: about 80 percent of visits to the doctor can be ascribed to stress-related complaints.

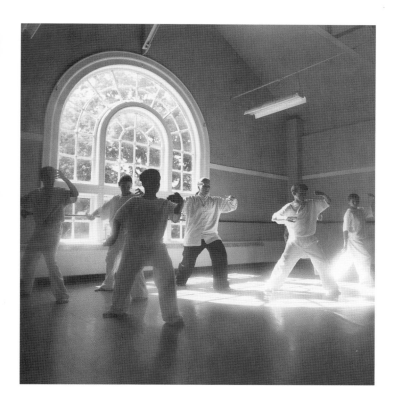

Eastern health practices seem to offer a route to inner peace as well as real health benefits. The holistic nature of Eastern systems—their emphasis on integrating the mind, body, and spirit—is ringing true for

■ A generation ago, few Westerners had the opportunity to learn tai chi—now there are classes suitable for young and old in almost every city.

more and more people. It now seems only common sense that we should treat the mind and the body as an indivisible whole.

And of course, tai chi is eminently suitable for a busy lifestyle. It can be fitted into any schedule—because all you need is a few minutes a day. Each practice will leave you feeling relaxed, as if a weight has been lifted. After a few sessions, you may start to notice changes in the way you stand and move. Eventually these changes will create lasting improvements to the way you feel. Tai chi is probably one of the most effective, health-enhancing ways to spend ten minutes.

About This Book

This book aims to tell you everything you need to know about establishing a tai chi practice at home. It can be used both by complete beginners and by more experienced practitioners.

The book is divided into sections. The first chapter gives the background to tai chi—what it is, why it works, and how it developed. The book goes on to look at the basic principles of the practice, including good posture and breathing. It then gives information on

■ *An introductory section at the beginning of the book explains the important ideas behind tai chi.*

Jargon-free text explains the important concepts

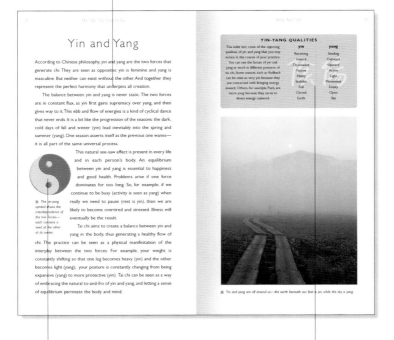

Color illustrations clarify the text

Useful information highlighted in boxes

how to learn tai chi and how to prepare for practice. It is essential to read these sections because they include important information on basic techniques and on safety.

The heart of the book is devoted to tai chi exercises, called the form. Each movement is clearly explained, and there is a color illustration to show you what to do at every step. The final section of the book explains how to integrate tai chi into your daily life.

Full-color picture with each step

Fair Lady Weaves the Shuttle (iv)

The final part of the sequence involves another turn of 270°, again in a clockwise direction. If you are finding it hard to work out which arm to raise, bear in mind that it is always the side with the leading leg.

1 Bring your weight onto the right leg, and turn your upper body to the right. Lift the left heel and turn the foot through a 90° angle to the right. Drop the left forearm, palm turning in. Lower the right arm, dropping the elbow and turning the palm to face you.

2 Now shift your weight onto the left leg, and continue to turn your body to the right. Lift the right heel and turn the foot to the right through a 90° angle. It should now point forward. Raise the right forearm, keeping the elbow low. Let the left forearm drop, turning the palm to face down. Your left fingers should point to the right hand.

3 Now bring your weight onto the right leg. Continue turning the upper body to the right. Lift the left heel and turn the foot through another 90° angle to the right.

4 Bring your weight onto the left leg. Move the right foot forward and to the right, in preparation for the bow and arrow stance. Keep turning your waist to the right. Letting your arms move with your upper body.

5 Continue the turn as you shift 70 per cent of your weight onto the right leg. Lift your left toes and turn the foot inward. Raise your right arm above your head, elbow bent and palm facing upward. The left arm moves forward, hand at shoulder level and palm facing outward. This ends the sequence.

Fair Lady Weaves the Shuttle (iv)

Each sequence is repeated on the next spread for quick reference

■ The entire tai chi form is explained, sequence by sequence, in easy-to-understand step text.

Tai chi is well-established as a safe form of exercise, and very few people experience any ill effects from doing it. However, if you are older, ill, or have a sedentary lifestyle, it is a good idea to check with your doctor before starting any new exercise. Tai chi movements should never cause strain or soreness. If the exercises feel awkward or result in any pain, stop and consult an experienced teacher.

■ *Simple exercises that apply the basic concepts of tai chi to everyday situations are given at the back of the book.*

Color photographs
accompany each step

In the Office

Working in an office can be bad for your health, especially if you sit at a computer. Office workers tend to remain in the same position for long periods, which can make the circulation sluggish. Get into the habit of checking your posture, and shift if you are uncomfortable. Get up and walk around every hour or so, and make sure that every day you find some time and a space to stretch out once a day.

ARM CIRCLES

Stand erect, feet hip width apart and arms by your sides. Sweep your hands to one side and then up over your head and down again in a large circular motion. Work gently and do not wrench or twist the body. Do this a couple of times in each direction. Repeat and the time bend your legs into a squat as your arms drop down. Do this twice in each direction. Breathe deeply as you exercise.

Keep the chest open
and relaxed

Knees slightly bent

Feet flat on floor

FOOT WORK

While sitting at your desk, take off your shoes and place the feet flat on the floor. Lift the heels up and hold for a moment, then return them to the floor and lift the balls and toes up. Do this five or six times, several times a day.

ARM SWINGS

Now turn your waist to one side, letting your arms follow the movement—taechi style—as you do so. Turn back to the front and then turn to the other side, again letting the arms follow. Do this for 30 seconds to one minute, breathing deeply. Work gently and do not force the movement farther than feels natural. Keep the knees slightly bent all the time.

FORWARD BEND

From a standing position, bend forward very slowly. Let your arms hang down. Keep the legs upright, knees slightly bent. Try to fold forward from the hips, letting the bend move slowly up the spine. Do not go any farther than is comfortable. To come up, bend your knees and slowly uncurl your spine from the base to the top. Lift your head up last.

Head drops down

Arms held out to the sides

SHAKE-OUT

Try the shake-out exercise to release tension and frustration. Stand in a relaxed tai chi posture. Bring your arms away from your body and gently shake them for a few moments. Bring all your weight onto one leg. Lift the other off the floor and shake it out. Then repeat with the other leg first in the standing position for a few minutes.

Boxes contain
useful reminders

Clear text explains
exactly what to do

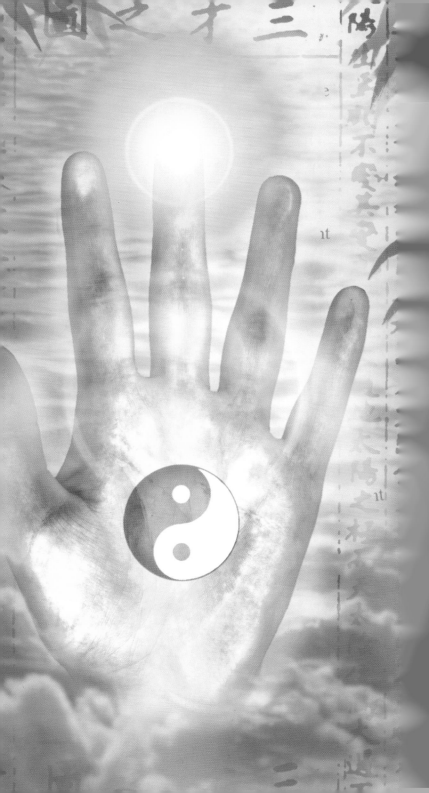

Why Tai Chi?

Tai chi was once only known in China. Today it is practiced all over the world. This section explores the ideas that lie at the center of this energizing health-giving system of exercise. And it looks at what the graceful art of tai chi can do for you.

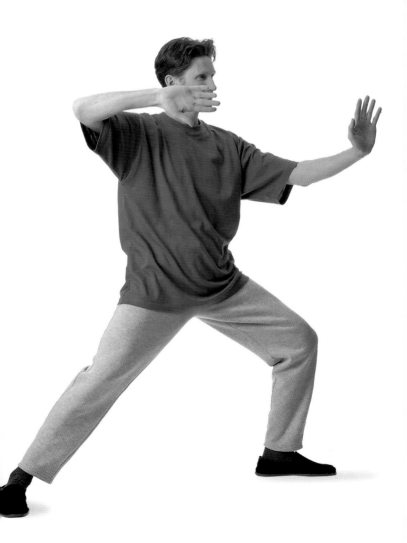

What is Tai Chi?

Tai chi is a gentle form of exercise that anyone can do. In China it is practiced daily by millions of people, old and young. And it is becoming increasingly popular in the West.

Tai chi is rooted in the theory that well-being depends on the circulation of life force (*chi*) around the body—the same idea lies behind acupuncture and other Eastern therapies. When chi becomes blocked or depleted, ill health or unhappiness are the result. Tai chi uses a combination of structured movements, deep breathing, and mental focus to enhance the flow of chi, thus promoting good health and helping to prevent illness.

The movements in tai chi are done gracefully and rhythmically—as though you are performing a dance (or a stylized fight) in slow motion. The actions appear very simple at first, but in fact it takes strength and awareness to maintain the degree of balance and muscular control demanded.

The movements are done in a strictly choreographed sequence, which is known as the form. The order never varies: tai chi practitioners, from the beginner to the master, do the same form. This element of repetition is key to tai chi because, once you know the basic moves, the only way to improve is to go deeper. The repetition does not become boring because tai chi engages the mind as well as the body. And there is always some element that can be improved upon—the flow of your breathing, the erectness of your posture, or the position of your hands.

What is more, tai chi is remarkably concise: once learned, the entire form takes about six minutes to perform. You need spend just a few minutes a day on tai chi, and very soon you will be reaping the benefits of this ancient and beautiful practice.

Tai chi is a way to build energy and strength within the body, which helps to maintain health and vigor.

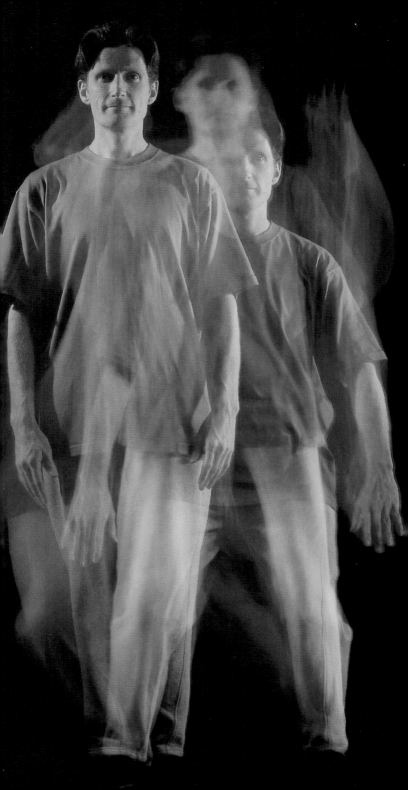

What Tai Chi Can Do for You

Tai chi is fantastically good for you. It is a holistic system, meaning that it benefits the mind and spirit as well as the physical body. Regular practice trains your powers of concentration, improves your mental awareness, and teaches you how to control stress.

The physical exercises combined with good breathing techniques help to improve your posture, flexibility, and balance. They also relax the muscles and nervous system, which in turn aids the functioning of the internal organs: practitioners claim that tai chi improves the digestion, lowers the blood pressure, and boosts the immune system.

Many of the benefits proceed from the slow, measured rhythm of tai chi. It is impossible to do tai chi in a frantic manner, and so it is impossible to remain stressed while you do it.

So many of the afflictions that plague Western society are due to the fact that we find it impossible to slow down and relax our minds and bodies. Tai chi is an orchestrated slowness, and that is its main strength. Simply watching a skilled practitioner doing tai chi can feel calming, and performing the movements brings a new sense of quietness to the mind and body.

As with acupuncture, nobody knows quite how tai chi works. Chi, the vital energy that all of us draw our strength from, is not detectable or quantifiable. We know that tai chi works because the people who do it attest to its benefits, some of which have now been backed up by scientific research. One US study found that tai chi improved breathing technique; another showed that it lowered blood pressure.

Of course, the benefits of tai chi come only if you do it regularly —all teachers stress the importance of establishing a daily practice. Getting into the habit of doing tai chi brings its own pleasure: it lets

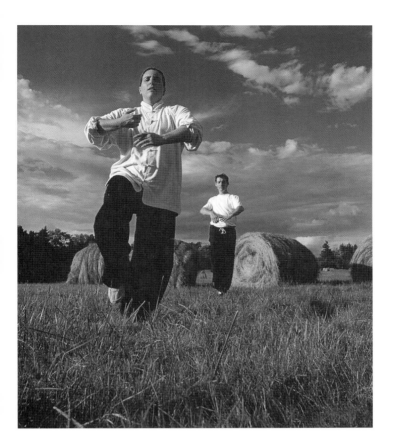

you earmark a short period each day in which you focus entirely on the needs of your body and mind—something that few of us remember to do in our daily lives.

Tai chi is good exercise for the body but it does not tire you out; you should feel energized after practice.

After a tai chi practice, you do not feel tired as you do after practicing other forms of exercise. Instead, you feel refreshed and alert. This is because tai chi builds and conserves energy in the body instead of expending it.

Many practitioners use tai chi as their only form of exercise. But although tai chi benefits the entire body, it does not work the heart and lungs in quite the same way as aerobic exercise. For this reason, it is ideally combined with regular brisk exercise, such as walking.

Where It All Began

The history of ancient things always consists of a mix of fact and myth. The harder you try to pin down a starting point, an original spark, the more myth and the less fact you are likely to encounter. This is especially true of tai chi, because the art was for many centuries practiced in secret. But what we can say for sure is that it originated in China, that it is related to other healing and martial arts such as chi kung and kung fu, and that it draws on the philosophy of Taoism.

Some time around 2700 B.C., the semi-mythological Yellow Emperor appears in a text that expounded on the invisible workings of the body, and gave rise to acupuncture. The Emperor is said to have practiced health-giving exercises based on the movements of animals. This is the first reference to something resembling chi kung or tai chi.

The Taoist thread in tai chi is older still. The core text of Taoism is the *I Ching, the Book of Changes*, written in about 2850 B.C. This is the first text to talk about chi (see *page 20*), yin and yang (see *page 22*). Lao Tzu, the Taoist sage, strove to explain the Tao (the "Way") in laconic epigrams. One of these could almost be a definition of tai chi: "Yield and overcome/ Bend and be straight/ He who stands on tiptoe is not steady/He who strides cannot maintain the pace."

A thousand year later, in the 6th century A.D., a Chinese physician named Hua-tuo taught exercises based on "the movement of the five creatures"—the bear, tiger, deer, ape, and bird. His system was called Wuchi chih hsi, and bears comparison with the Yellow Emperor's regime: both were based on observations of nature, and both were intended primarily as a health-giving practice.

Around the same time, an Indian monk named Bodhidharma brought Zen Buddhism to China. He taught the monks at the Shaolin temple at Henan, and invented a series of exercises to help strengthen mind and body for meditation. These exercises—called Shaolin

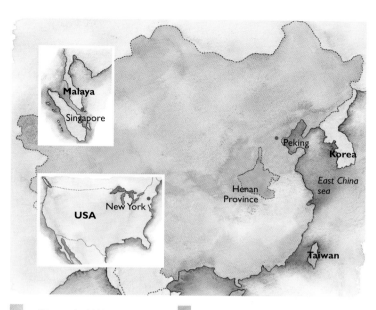

China in the 1800s   Henan, birthplace of tai chi

THE HISTORY

The origins of tai chi could go back as far as 5,000 years, but the form as we know it today did not emerge until the 13th century.

2700 B.C.

The Yellow Emperor, the father of Chinese medicine, practices exercises based on movements of animals

6th century A.D.

Bodhidharma, founder of Zen Buddhism, teaches mind-body exercises to monks at Shaolin temple in Henan.

13th century

Chang San Feng devises early system of tai chi, after seeing a snake and crane fighting

18th century

Chen family of Henan practice tai chi in secret

1800s

Yang Lu-chan learns Chen style. He goes on to develop and teach Yang style.

1880s

Chinese emigrants spread tai chi to Singapore.

1930s

Cheng Man-ching trains with Yang Chen-fu, grandson of Yang Lu-chan

1940s

Cheng Man-ching simplifies Yang style into short form, now the most widely practiced style in the world.

1949

Cheng Man-ching moves to Taiwan, where he opens a school in Taipei

1960s

Tai chi starts to become popular in the West. Cheng Man-ching opens a school in New York

boxing—developed into the martial art we know as kung fu. One of those to learn martial arts at Shaolin was Chang San Feng, who was born in 1247. He is usually said to be the true founder of tai chi chuan, as it came to be known. The name is untranslatable but might be rendered as the "great strength of opposites."

Chang San Feng's eureka moment was the result of a chance encounter—and once again the inspiration came from the animal world. Chang is said to have seen a fight between a crane and a snake. Neither could overcome the other: the snake could twist out of reach of the bird's beak; the bird could step aside from the snake's lunges, or disperse their power with his wings. Chang developed a martial art that was based on giving way to force, bending with the blow.

Some time during the medieval Ming dynasty, tai chi became the secret monopoly of the Chen clan, and was taught only to members of the family. This exclusive arrangement was broken in the 19th century by a servant of the Chens. Yang Lu-chan learned the art and went on to teach an adapted form—Yang-style tai chi—to the courtiers of the Ching Emperor.

Tai chi was brought out of China in the 20th century. One of the teachers who did most to spread tai chi worldwide was Cheng Man-ching, who fled to Taiwan after the communist revolution in 1947. Cheng Man-ching was a kind of renaissance man of Chinese wisdom and an expert in herbal medicine. He used his tai chi to control his tuberculosis, and put the emphasis on the therapeutic qualities of the practice. He also invented a "short form" which, by the time he died in 1975, had spread to the West.

■ *The monk Chang San Feng is credited as the founder of tai chi. But nobody really knows whether he existed or not.*

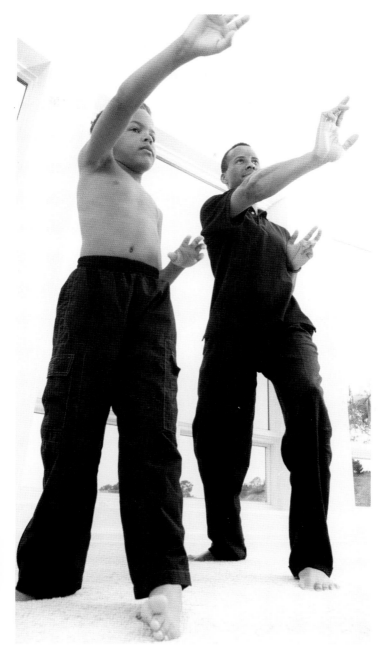

Tai chi was once the preserve of a select few. It is now practiced by ordinary people all over the world, thanks largely to Cheng Man-ching and his accessible short form.

What is Chi?

It is notoriously difficult to explain what chi is. The idea of a universal life force, an ineluctable energy that bathes the universe and flows through all living things, is alien to Western science. Chi is literally indefinable in English. All one can say is that chi seems to be akin to the well-understood force of electricity in that it flows, it is invisible, and it is present in the body.

Chi is the central idea of Chinese medicine—and of the Eastern understanding of the world. It is seen as the vital, animating force that gives life to all things and upon which our mental, physical, and spiritual health depends. The therapeutic practices of acupuncture are based on directing the flow of chi (or *qi*, as the word is sometimes transcribed) to wherever it is needed. In Japan, chi is called *ki*, and here too it is manipulated as a way of maintaining good health. Practitioners of Indian yoga also know this energy, which they call *prana*.

Tai chi, like yoga, is a means of gathering and managing life energy. This control is possible because chi, which we draw in with our breath, runs down fixed channels or meridians in the body. The subtle movements of the tai chi form are designed to regulate the flow of chi—speeding it here, slowing it there, and removing blockages in its path.

Tai chi also aims to store chi in the body. The main storehouse is the lower tan tien, which is just below the navel. Tai chi practitioners say that all the movements of the form proceed from this tan tien: they draw on its strength and at the same time they build its power.

As you learn tai chi, you will become increasingly aware of these processes. You will be able to feel the chi flowing and growing within you. This is one of the aims and the pleasures of tai chi practice.

■ *Tai chi philosophy states that there are three main centers of energy in the body. These are known as tan tiens, and the most important one lies just below the navel.*

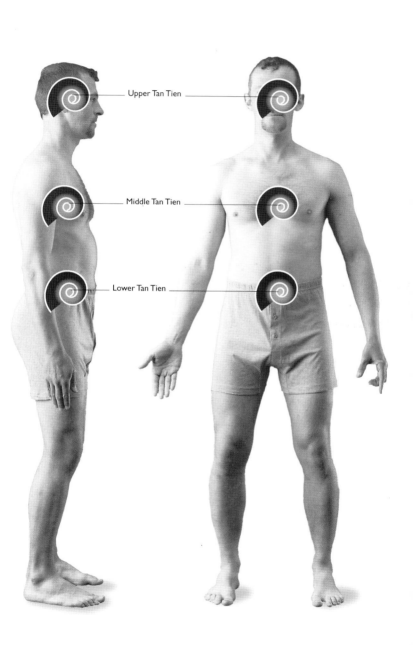

Upper Tan Tien

Middle Tan Tien

Lower Tan Tien

Yin and Yang

According to Chinese philosophy, yin and yang are the two forces that generate chi. They are seen as opposites: yin is feminine and yang is masculine. But neither can exist without the other. And together they represent the perfect harmony that underpins all creation.

The balance between yin and yang is never static. The two forces are in constant flux, as yin first gains supremacy over yang, and then gives way to it. This ebb and flow of energies is a kind of cyclical dance that never ends. It is a bit like the progression of the seasons: the dark, cold days of fall and winter (yin) lead inevitably into the spring and summer (yang). One season asserts itself as the previous one wanes—it is all part of the same universal process.

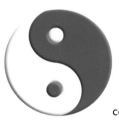

■ *The yin-yang symbol shows the interdependence of the two forces— each contains a seed of the other at its center.*

This natural see-saw effect is present in every life and in each person's body. An equilibrium between yin and yang is essential to happiness and good health. Problems arise if one force dominates for too long. So, for example, if we continue to be busy (activity is seen as yang) when really we need to pause (rest is yin), then we are likely to become overtired and stressed. Illness will eventually be the result.

Tai chi aims to create a balance between yin and yang in the body, thus generating a healthy flow of chi. The practice can be seen as a physical manifestation of the interplay between the two forces. For example, your weight is constantly shifting so that one leg becomes heavy (yin) and the other becomes light (yang); your posture is constantly changing from being expansive (yang) to more protective (yin). Tai chi can be seen as a way of embracing the natural to-and-fro of yin and yang, and letting a sense of equilibrium permeate the body and mind.

YIN-YANG QUALITIES

The table lists some of the opposing qualities of yin and yang that you may notice in the course of your practice. You can see the forces of yin and yang at work in different postures of tai chi. Some stances such as Rollback can be seen as very yin because they are concerned with bringing energy inward. Others, for example Push, are more yang because they serve to direct energy outward.

yin	yang
Receiving	Sending
Inward	Outward
Downward	Upward
Passive	Active
Heavy	Light
Stability	Movement
Full	Empty
Closed	Open
Earth	Sky

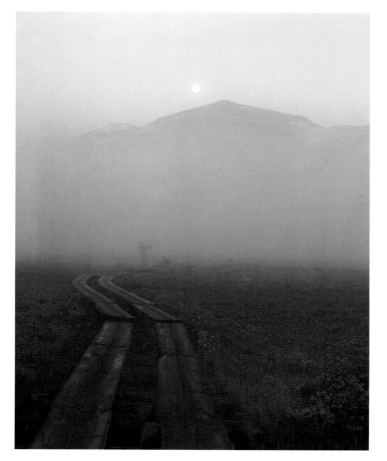

■ Yin and yang are all around us—the earth beneath our feet is yin, while the sky is yang.

A World of Energy

Tai chi is traditionally done outdoors, where you can garner fresh chi from the clean air. If you go to China, you will see groups of people doing their daily practice in parks. But you do not have to subscribe to the notion of chi to benefit from taking your exercise out doors, and, of course, you do not have to do your tai chi outdoors at all if you do not want to.

Nevertheless, there are real benefits to be had from doing your tai chi under an open sky. Practicing outside can strengthen your connection with the natural environment. As you develop the meditative state of mind that tai chi requires, you will automatically imbibe a deeper understanding of your place in the universe.

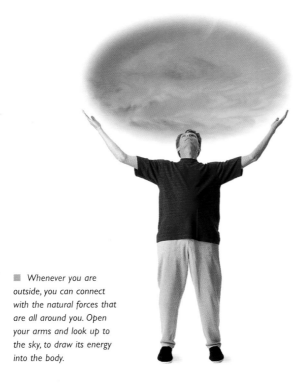

■ *Whenever you are outside, you can connect with the natural forces that are all around you. Open your arms and look up to the sky, to draw its energy into the body.*

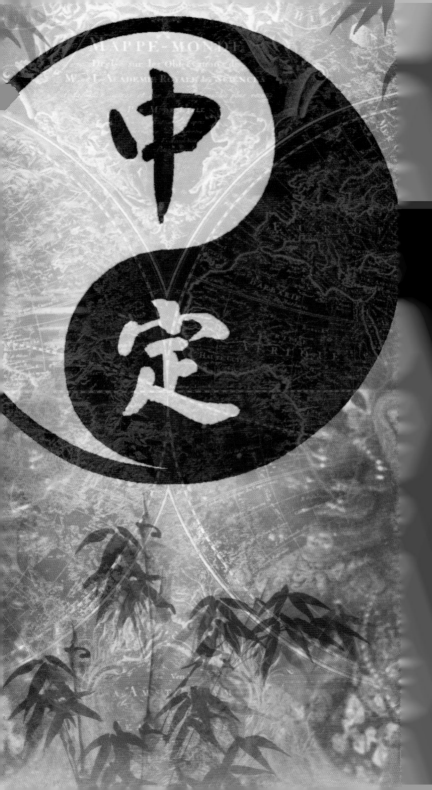

Principles of Practice

Tai chi works on all aspects of the self—the mind, body, and spirit. This chapter looks at the different elements involved in tai chi, from posture to mental focus. It includes exercises to help you develop your understanding of these elements and put them into practice.

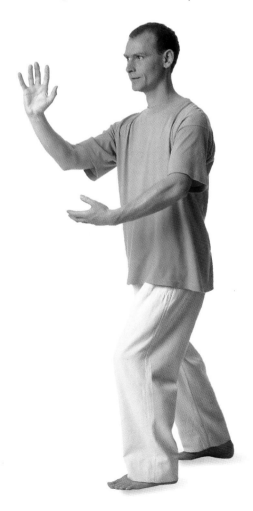

Posture

Good posture is an essential element of tai chi. The many movements involved mean you have to pay constant attention to how you hold yourself. Over time you will become aware of the alignment of your joints, and you will learn to keep your muscles relaxed even while you are moving. But first you need to stand in the correct tai chi way.

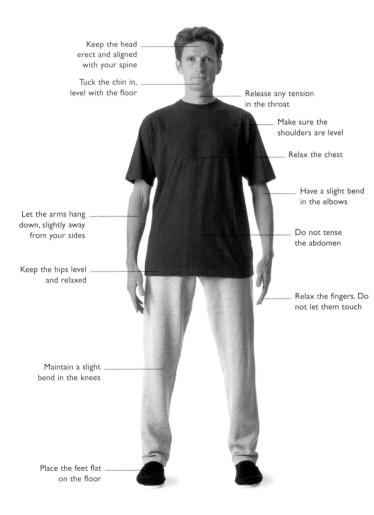

Keep the head erect and aligned with your spine

Tuck the chin in, level with the floor

Release any tension in the throat

Make sure the shoulders are level

Relax the chest

Have a slight bend in the elbows

Let the arms hang down, slightly away from your sides

Do not tense the abdomen

Keep the hips level and relaxed

Relax the fingers. Do not let them touch

Maintain a slight bend in the knees

Place the feet flat on the floor

RELAX THE BACK

Try to release tension in the back and shoulders. Your shoulder blades should be drawn in and downward. The spine should be erect but relaxed. Imagine it is hanging down, as though supported by a cord that is attached to the top of your head. It will help if you keep your tail bone (coccyx) and chin tucked in.

Shoulder blades are
drawn downward

Spine is erect, in line
with the head

Tail bone is tucked in

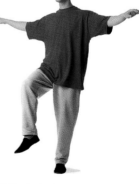

■ *Tai chi develops your balance so that you maintain good posture even when standing on one leg.*

Sinking Your Weight

Tai chi teachers often talk about dropping your weight downward. This can be a difficult concept to grasp when you start learning tai chi. It is partly to do with releasing tension in the upper body, which should feel light, and it also involves keeping your knees bent, so that you are physically closer to the ground. But sinking down is also a mental process—you have to imagine the weight dropping down through your legs and into the ground below.

SINKING EXERCISE

Stand in the tai chi way, following the checklist on the previous pages. Bend your knees, so that you lower yourself by an inch or two. Your legs should immediately feel heavier. Take care you do not tense the abdomen: bring your hands in front of your belly and try to relax here as you let your legs take your weight. Do this for a minute, then come up slowly.

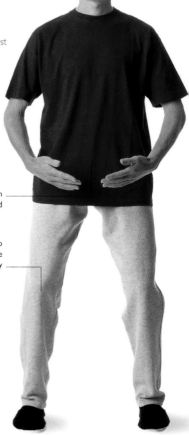

Keep the abdomen soft and relaxed

Bend the knees to help absorb the weight of your body

KEEPING LOW

You should keep sinking down throughout a tai chi practice. Be sure that you sink into the final posture of each sequence before moving on to the next one. This will help you to gain the full benefits of each pose.

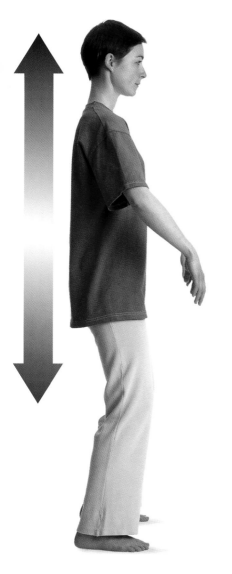

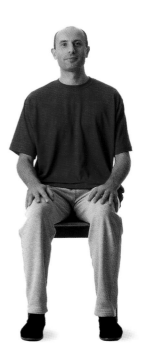

SITTING EXERCISE

Practice tai chi posture whenever you have a few moments to spare. You can practice some elements when sitting down: keep your feet flat on the floor, toes forward, and rest your hands on your thighs. Keep the upper body relaxed but erect as you imagine your weight sinking down, through the coccyx into the ground.

EXTENDING THE SPINE

When you sink your weight down, take care that you do not slouch or slump the upper body. Keep your spine erect—think of it as connecting you with both the sky and the earth. The top of the spine extends upward, as you relax the shoulders and tuck in the chin. The base of the spine drops downward, as you tuck in the tail bone.

Movement

You are constantly moving in tai chi. Each sequence in the form leads seamlessly into the next, creating one continuous flow. But tai chi also incorporates an element of stillness. You begin and end the form standing quietly for a short period. And as you complete each sequence, you pause for the briefest of moments and sink into the final posture before you move on to the next one. The movements of tai chi are never forced or rushed. Instead, they are performed in a slow, seemingly effortless way. For this reason, tai chi is often described as "meditation in motion."

To an observer, it may look as though the arms work very hard in tai chi. In fact, all your movements emanate from the energy center (tan tien) in the abdominal region. You never simply extend your arm out—the action unfolds from the core of the body and is coordinated with the turning of the waist. As you practice tai chi, you will see that the legs, too, follow the turns of the waist. This is what gives the movements their characteristic flow.

Stability is the key to performing the actions slowly and with control. In tai chi, there are many subtle shifts in the position of the feet and the balance of your weight. These are designed to root you to the ground, so that you are like a tree which sways in the wind but stays in touch with the earth.

■ *The movements of tai chi unfold in an effortless flow. Start each action from your waist and let it travel through your body.*

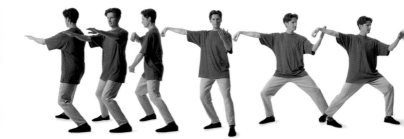

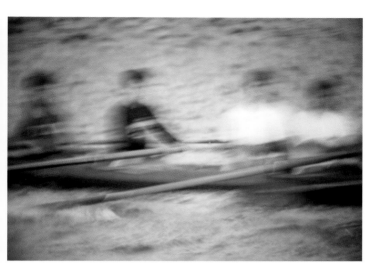

The motion of a row boat depends on all the oarsmen moving in synchronization. In the same way, movement in tai chi depends on all parts of the body working in harmony.

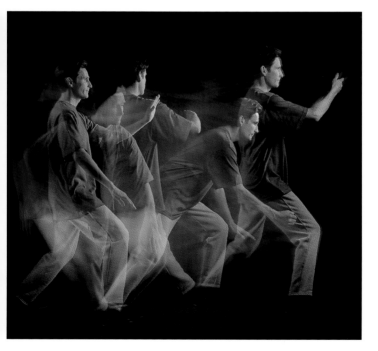

Tai chi is practiced slowly. Try to develop a steady pace, so that each movement is performed at the same speed. This will help bring grace and rhythm to your practice.

Breathing

In tai chi, your breathing is as slow as your movements. Keep the mouth closed and breathe through the nostrils. Take long deep inhalations, and exhale for the same length of time. Be sure to keep your breathing quiet—like the actions, it should never be forced or rushed. As you become more practiced in learning tai chi, your breathing may start to harmonize with the movements.

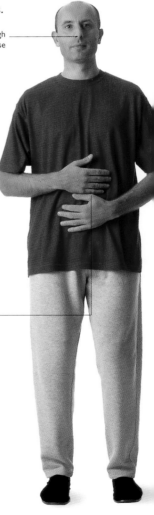

Breathe through the nose

ABDOMINAL BREATHING

Children naturally practice the deep, relaxed abominal breathing that is used in tai chi. If you watch a baby breathe, you will see how its abdomen rises with the inhalation and falls with the exhalation. As we grow up, most of us develop poor breathing habits. We start to take shallow breaths, particularly when under stress. This reduces the amount of oxygen that gets into the blood—which in turn affects our energy levels and well-being. The following exercise will help you to develop your awareness of abdominal breathing.

Feel your abdomen rise and fall with your breath

I Stand tall, in the tai chi posture. Place your hands on your abdomen: one should rest on your navel; the other just below it. The lower hand is on your tan tien, the body's main energy store. Breathe for a minute or two, and simply notice whether your hands rise and fall as you breathe in and out.

HOW WE BREATHE

The mechanical process of breathing is controlled by the combined action of the diaphragm and the tiny muscles between the ribs. They work together to expand and contract the chest cavity, which changes the air pressure inside it. This has the effect of drawing air into the body (inhalation), or forcing it out (exhalation).

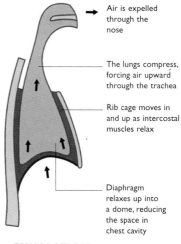

Air rushes into the nostrils, then passes down the trachea into lungs

Trachea (windpipe)

Intercostal muscles contract, causing the rib cage to move out and down

The diaphragm flattens creating more space in the chest cavity

INHALATION

Air is expelled through the nose

The lungs compress, forcing air upward through the trachea

Rib cage moves in and up as intercostal muscles relax

Diaphragm relaxes up into a dome, reducing the space in chest cavity

EXHALATION

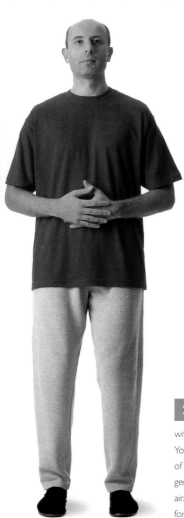

2 Now imagine that the air you breathe is filling your abdomen. Feel your hands rise with the inhalation and fall with the exhalation. You may find it helpful to rest one hand on top of the other. As you exhale, press the area gently inward—as though helping to expel the air. Release the pressure as you inhale. Do this for a couple of minutes at a time.

Mental Awareness

Tai chi works on both mind and body. You will find that it is impossible to practice the exercises properly if you are thinking about something else. You need to be fully aware of what you are doing in order to maintain right posture and balance. When you start to practice tai chi, all your attention will be on remembering and coordinating the actions. It is a good idea to practice each sequence several times so that you are familiar with them before going on to the next one.

Once you know the steps, you can expand your mental awareness to encompass deeper elements of the practice. It is like being a musician—first you learn the notes, then you learn to play them in a way that is meaningful rather than merely mechanical. You may find it helps to concentrate on a different aspect of tai chi each day—for example, relaxing the shoulders, practicing abdominal breathing, or letting your movements unfold from the abdomen. Sometimes, you may like to focus on bringing a spirit of joyfulness to the practice. Eventually, all these elements will meld into a harmonious whole.

One important thing is to make sure that you direct your attention to each movement as you make it. It is said that chi follows the mind—in other words, energy goes to the place you are thinking about. If you imagine your hand rising up, you may find that it seems to move without effort. This is the effect of chi.

Don't worry if you find it hard to stay focused; just keep bringing your attention gently back to what you are doing. With regular practice your powers of concentration will improve.

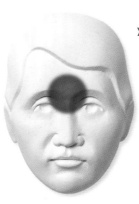

■ *The power of your mind is concentrated in the upper tan tien or third eye. Use it to direct your movements and the flow of chi around your body.*

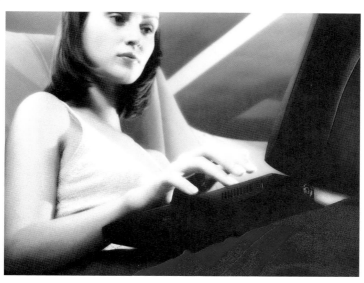

■ We are used to concentrating in our daily lives, but we rarely harmonize mind and body in the way that tai chi lets us do.

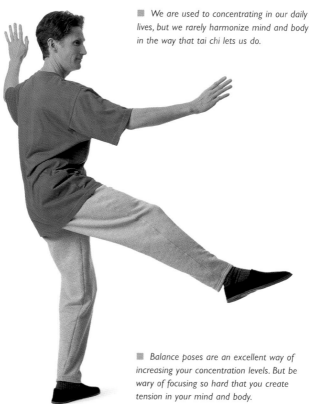

■ Balance poses are an excellent way of increasing your concentration levels. But be wary of focusing so hard that you create tension in your mind and body.

Practicing Stepping

It is a good idea to practice bringing the principles of tai chi to a few
basic movements before you move on to the form. In this exercise,
you start from a good standing posture and simply step to the side.
You may find it helpful to focus on maintaining good posture at first.
Then, start to incorporate the other elements of the practice, one by
one, as you continue to step from one foot to the other.

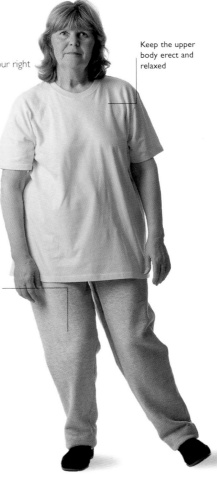

Keep the upper
body erect and
relaxed

1 Bring all your weight onto your right
leg. Lift up your left foot and
move it out to the side. The space
between your feet should be
equivalent to the distance
between the outer edges of
your shoulders—one shoulder-
width. Place the inner side gently
on the ground, toes pointing
forward, then roll down the rest
of the foot. Do not start to put
any weight on it until it is flat on
the ground.

All your weight should be
on the supporting leg

ABSORBING THE WEIGHT

As you shift your weight
from one leg to the other,
bend the supporting knee
well—this helps to absorb
the weight. The other leg will
start to straighten, but keep
a slight bend in the knee.

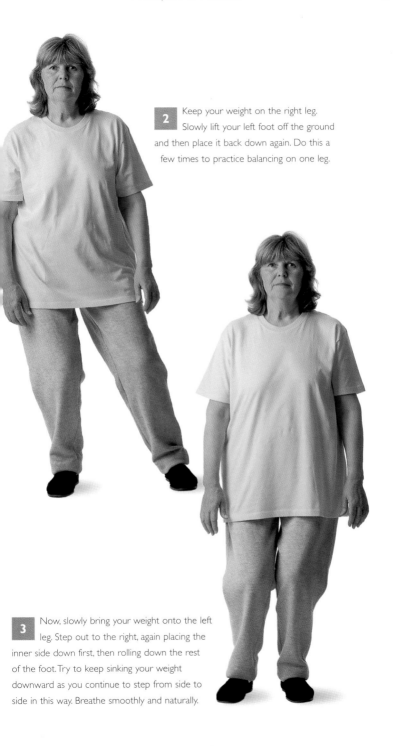

2 Keep your weight on the right leg. Slowly lift your left foot off the ground and then place it back down again. Do this a few times to practice balancing on one leg.

3 Now, slowly bring your weight onto the left leg. Step out to the right, again placing the inner side down first, then rolling down the rest of the foot. Try to keep sinking your weight downward as you continue to step from side to side in this way. Breathe smoothly and naturally.

Basic Stances

The same foot positions are often repeated in the tai chi form. You usually step into one of the basic stances shown here. Try practicing each stance several times, so that you are familiar with it before you start to learn the form. Remember to keep sinking your weight downward. Repeat each stance on both sides—so that you step out with the left foot as well as the right.

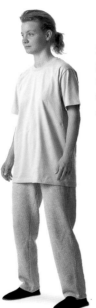

PARALLEL STANCE

Stand with your feet together, toes pointing forward. Bring your weight into the left leg, then lift up the right one and move it out to the side. Place the foot down, heel first, so that the feet are parallel and about one shoulder-width apart. This position first appears at the start of the form.

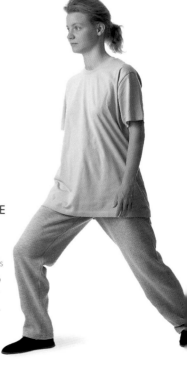

BOW AND ARROW STANCE

Start in parallel stance. Lift the left toes, and turn the foot outward through a 45° angle. Place the foot flat. Bring your weight onto this leg. Lift up the right foot and step forward, so that there is a distance between your feet of about one and a half times the width of your shoulders. Bring most of your weight onto the right leg, and bend the knee.

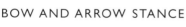

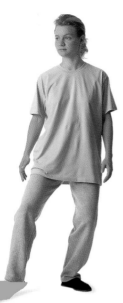

TOE OR CAT STANCE

Stand with your feet together. Lift the left toes and turn the heel outward through a 90° angle. Place the foot flat, and bring most of your weight onto this leg. Raise the right foot and step forward, keeping your weight back. Place the foot so that it is at right angles to the left one. Rest only the ball of your foot on the floor, and keep the heel lifted. Most of your weight remains on the back leg.

WIDE STANCE

This stance is similar to the bow and arrow stance, but your feet are at right angles to each other. From parallel stance, lift the left toes and turn the heel out through 90°. Place the foot down flat, and bring most of your weight onto this leg. Step forward with the right foot. Place the heel down first, at right angles to the left one. The distance between your feet should be equal to one and a half times your shoulder width.

HEEL STANCE

This is the same as the toe or cat stance, but this time you place the heel of the right foot on the floor and leave the toes and ball raised. Make sure that you do not straighten the right leg—the knee should remain slightly bent.

Tai Chi Walking

Once you have mastered the basic steps, try tai chi walking. This gets you used to moving the legs while keeping the upper body erect. It is also a good meditation exercise, which you can practice whenever you need to slow down. Mark out an area of 33 feet, in a large room or outside. Walk to the end, then pause and check your posture. Turn around and walk back the other way. Do this for about ten minutes.

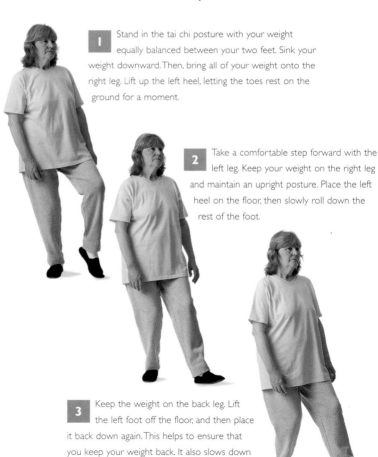

1 Stand in the tai chi posture with your weight equally balanced between your two feet. Sink your weight downward. Then, bring all of your weight onto the right leg. Lift up the left heel, letting the toes rest on the ground for a moment.

2 Take a comfortable step forward with the left leg. Keep your weight on the right leg and maintain an upright posture. Place the left heel on the floor, then slowly roll down the rest of the foot.

3 Keep the weight on the back leg. Lift the left foot off the floor, and then place it back down again. This helps to ensure that you keep your weight back. It also slows down the movement. Keep your breathing deep and relaxed as you step.

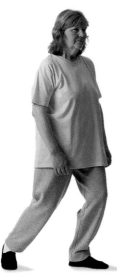

4 Now slowly bring your weight onto the left leg. As you do this, bend the left knee and let the right one straighten slightly—keep it soft. Keep your posture upright; do not start to lean forward.

5 When all of your weight is on the left leg, step forward with the right foot. Again, place the heel down first and then roll the rest of the foot onto the floor. Keep the weight on the back leg and raise the right foot to check your balance, then put it down again.

Let your arms hang down by your sides, without touching

6 Continue to step forward. Make sure that you always transfer your weight onto the supporting leg before you take a step. You may also like to try walking backward in a similar way. When stepping backward. always place the toes of the leading foot on the ground first, instead of your heel.

Moving the Upper Body

This sequence, called Rollback, is taken from the tai chi form. It is a good exercise to practice moving the arms as you turn the waist and shift your weight. The feet are in the bow and arrow stance, with the left foot forward and the right behind. They remain in this position throughout the sequence. Do the exercise several times, coordinating the actions of your arms with the turns of the waist. Then change position so that the right leg is forward, and repeat on the other side.

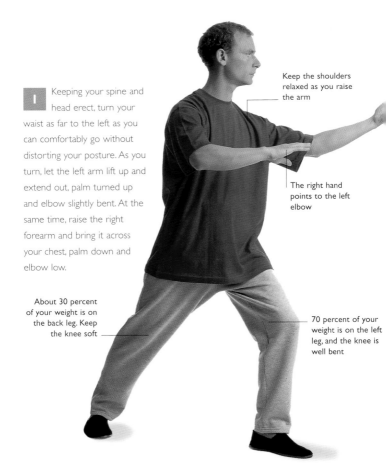

1 Keeping your spine and head erect, turn your waist as far to the left as you can comfortably go without distorting your posture. As you turn, let the left arm lift up and extend out, palm turned up and elbow slightly bent. At the same time, raise the right forearm and bring it across your chest, palm down and elbow low.

Keep the shoulders relaxed as you raise the arm

The right hand points to the left elbow

About 30 percent of your weight is on the back leg. Keep the knee soft

70 percent of your weight is on the left leg, and the knee is well bent

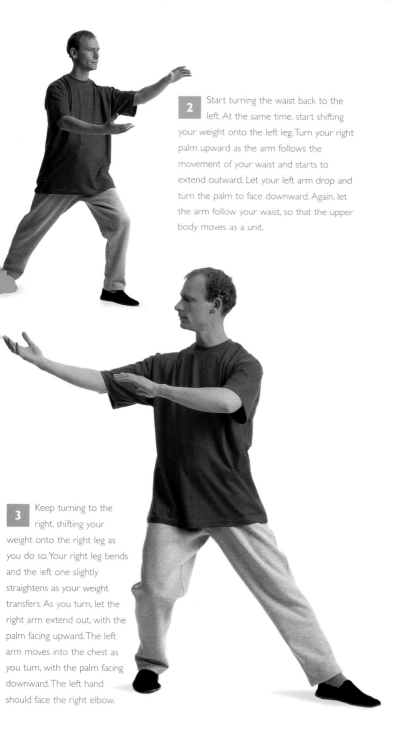

2 Start turning the waist back to the left. At the same time, start shifting your weight onto the left leg. Turn your right palm upward as the arm follows the movement of your waist and starts to extend outward. Let your left arm drop and turn the palm to face downward. Again, let the arm follow your waist, so that the upper body moves as a unit.

3 Keep turning to the right, shifting your weight onto the right leg as you do so. Your right leg bends and the left one slightly straightens as your weight transfers. As you turn, let the right arm extend out, with the palm facing upward. The left arm moves into the chest as you turn, with the palm facing downward. The left hand should face the right elbow.

Developing the Practice

Tai chi teachers say that you can learn tai chi in just a few months—but that it takes a lifetime to master it. In this respect, tai chi is rather like learning a language: you can quickly get a grasp on the basics, but it takes years to become fluent. To put it another way, tai chi is both easy and difficult. However good you become, there are always subtle improvements you can make, new challenges for you to face.

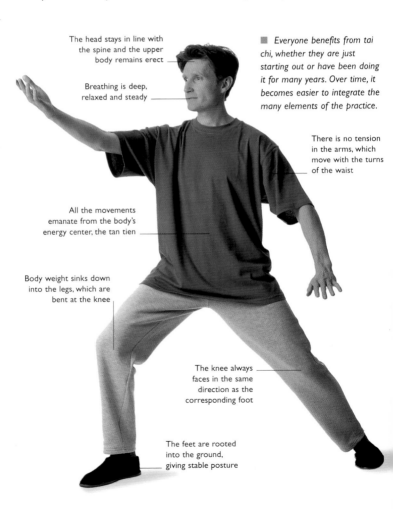

The head stays in line with the spine and the upper body remains erect

Breathing is deep, relaxed and steady

■ *Everyone benefits from tai chi, whether they are just starting out or have been doing it for many years. Over time, it becomes easier to integrate the many elements of the practice.*

There is no tension in the arms, which move with the turns of the waist

All the movements emanate from the body's energy center, the tan tien

Body weight sinks down into the legs, which are bent at the knee

The knee always faces in the same direction as the corresponding foot

The feet are rooted into the ground, giving stable posture

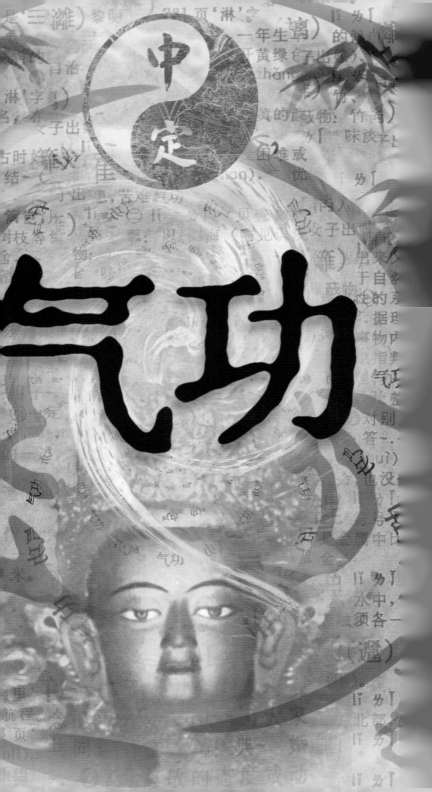

Getting Started

You can practice tai chi anywhere and at any time. There is no need for any special equipment, and you do not have to spend very long on your practice—just a few minutes a day is enough to gain the benefits of this ancient art. However, you will get more out of your tai chi if you do it regularly, and if you try to practice at the same time each day. This chapter gives some advice on how to learn tai chi and make the most of practicing at home. It tells you what you should wear and how you should prepare for a tai chi session with a few warming-up exercises. There are also some exercises that show you how to build and conserve energy in the body. These are taken from chi kung, a discipline that is related to tai chi and often taught with it.

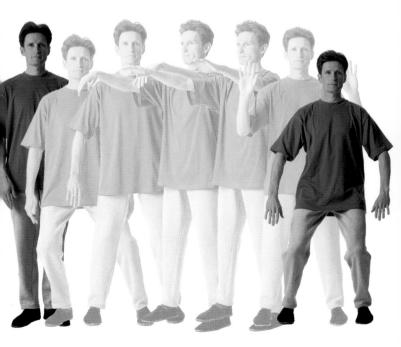

Learning Tai Chi

Anyone can learn tai chi. All you need do is to set aside a few minutes each day in order to memorize and practice the sequences.

Most teachers would say that learning tai chi, like practicing tai chi, is something that should be done slowly. This means concentrating on one or two sequences at a time. Ideally you should be fully familiar with one sequence before you try to assimilate the next. Little by little, you will get to know the form.

To learn a new sequence, read all the directions before you start. You will almost certainly need to look at the directions again—it can be helpful to prop the book up somewhere you can see it. You might like to learn with a friend, so that you can take it in turns to read the instructions out loud. You could also record them on a tape recorder—in which case you should speak very slowly. Most people need to practice the sequence several times before they remember it.

When you are doing tai chi, it is important that you start right at the beginning of the form, and then add new sequences to your repertoire as you go. It is like learning a poem by heart: it does not make sense if you know the lines in wrong order. So, always follow the time-hallowed sequence of the form. Do not try to rush through— the quality of the practice is more important than the number of sequences that you know.

If you can, go to classes. Meeting other people interested in tai chi will help your motivation. More importantly, a teacher will be able to guide you through the many nuances of the form. He or she will also be able to correct your habitual errors. For example, perhaps you have a tendency to raise your shoulders whenever you move your arms or perhaps you are holding your breath when you take a step or do a complicated action. A teacher will help you to develop and refine your practice, so that you can enjoy it at a deeper level.

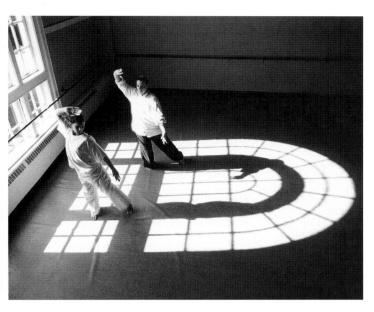

■ *Working with a partner can help you to stay motivated. Practice synchronizing your movements—as though you are performing the same dance.*

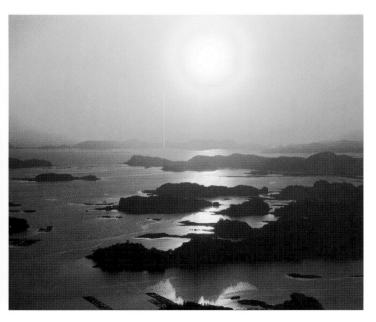

■ *Tai chi is traditionally practiced twice a day, at sunrise and sunset. It can be a wonderful way to start and end your day, particularly if you practice outside.*

Guidelines for Practice

Tai chi practitioners often exercise early in the morning and again in the early evening. You should choose a regular time that fits in with your schedule—it doesn't matter when you practice as long as you do. Try to establish a routine and stick to it.

These guidelines will help you get the most from your practice.

● Practice little and often. Try to do tai chi for at least ten minutes every day. You can practice for an hour or more if you like, but do not do so much that you become tired. As you become more adept, you may like to add another session later in the day.

● Always do tai chi in a quiet space. It is good to practise outdoors; otherwise use a peaceful, tidy room in your home. Ask anyone you live with to leave you alone while you do your tai chi. Turn off any phones.

● Wear loose, comfortable clothing that does not restrict your movements. Tracksuit pants and a loose T-shirt are ideal; add a sweat shirt if it is cold. The Chinese wear special thin-soled shoes for tai chi—you can buy these in Chinese stores or you can use a pair of light canvas shoes.

■ *Always wear shoes when practicing tai chi —make sure that they have thin soles that bend with your feet.*

● Do not eat a large amount just before practicing tai chi, wait three hours after a heavy meal.

● Be in a calm frame of mind. If you are feeling stressed, angry, or upset, sit quietly and breathe for a few minutes first. You may also find it helpful to go for a walk to release physical tension from your body before you start your tai chi.

● Always warm up the body with a few simple exercises. There are some exercises given in this chapter, but you can develop your own routine if you prefer. Always warm up very gently, and avoid jerky movements. Breathe deeply as you warm up.

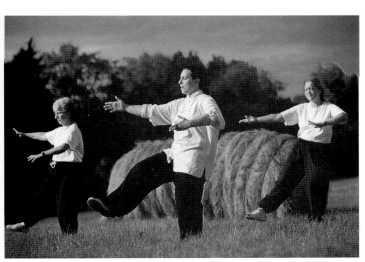

■ There is more chi outside in the countryside and parks than indoors or in built-up areas. Practicing tai chi outdoors will draw fresh energy into the body.

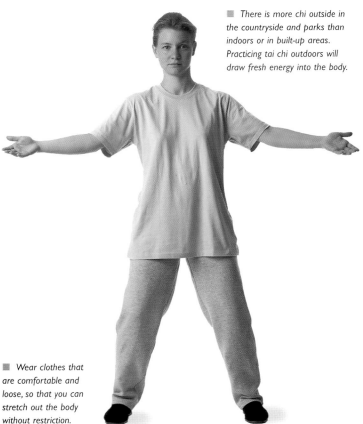

■ Wear clothes that are comfortable and loose, so that you can stretch out the body without restriction.

Warming Up

You should always warm up the body before practicing tai chi. You can use any exercises you like to do this, but be sure to stretch the arms and legs, and mobilize the joints. Stand in a relaxed posture to start.

In tai chi, you frequently turn the waist from right to left and back again. It is therefore a good idea to begin warming up with some waist turns. This helps you to limber up, and it also reminds you right from the start about the importance of the body's center in tai chi.

To practice waist turns, place your hands on your hips and turn the upper body to one side. Turn back to the front, then round to the other side. Repeat a few times, turning only as far as is comfortable. As you turn, direct your attention to the lower abdomen: focus on the area an inch below your navel—your tan tien.

NECK STRETCH

Release tension in the neck with a few stretches. Be very gentle—never force the neck farther than it naturally goes.

1 Stand in tai chi posture. Lift the shoulders up toward your ears, then let them drop. Do this a few times. Now, slowly turn your head to the right. Return to the front, then turn to the left. Do this a few times.

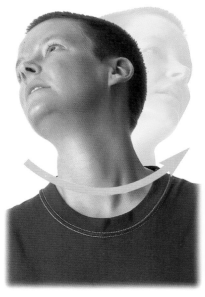

2 Drop the head sidewise to the right. Bring up to the center, then drop to the left. Do this a few times. Now, lift your chin up and to the side in a looping action. Curve it back down, then—up to the other side—following an arc. Repeat the action a few times.

SHAKING OUT

Try a quick and gentle shake-out to release tension in the body, and warm up the muscles. This exercise helps to stimulate your circulation and encourage the free flow of energy around the body. Work from the feet upward.

1 Start by standing up in a relaxed posture, feet hip-width apart. Raise one leg and gently shake the foot. Let the shake encompass the whole leg. Repeat on the other side.

2 Lift your arms away from the body and shake the hands. Expand the action to shake the arms. Then start to move the whole body very gently from side to side, back to front—legs, arms, hips, waist, torso, and head. Bend the knees up and down as you shake very gently.

Let the whole arm move as one

Keep the leg muscles relaxed as you shake

IMPORTANT

Don't be tempted to skip the warming up—you will get more out of the tai chi form if your body is relaxed when you start. Warming up also helps you to prepare mentally—use the time to set aside any worries.

Warming Up

Here are some good exercises to stretch out the limbs. They also
work to mobilize the hips and shoulders. Use a wall for support if you
find it hard to keep your balance during the leg exercise.

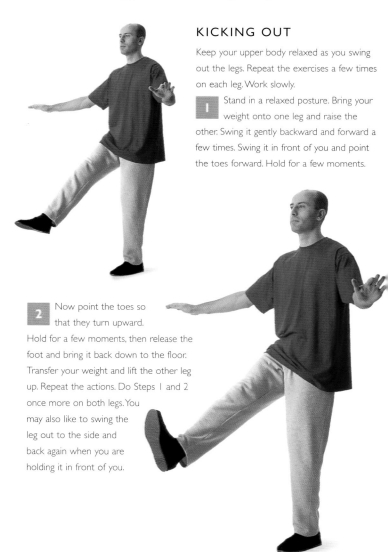

KICKING OUT

Keep your upper body relaxed as you swing
out the legs. Repeat the exercises a few times
on each leg. Work slowly.

1 Stand in a relaxed posture. Bring your
weight onto one leg and raise the
other. Swing it gently backward and forward a
few times. Swing it in front of you and point
the toes forward. Hold for a few moments.

2 Now point the toes so
that they turn upward.
Hold for a few moments, then release the
foot and bring it back down to the floor.
Transfer your weight and lift the other leg
up. Repeat the actions. Do Steps 1 and 2
once more on both legs. You
may also like to swing the
leg out to the side and
back again when you are
holding it in front of you.

LIFTING UP

These exercises help to expand the chest and lungs, and they also loosen your shoulder joints. Breathe deeply.

1 Stand in a relaxed posture. Lift up the arms, bending the elbows and keeping the palms turned in. Raise the arms above your head and look up. Lower your arms, bring them out and down in a arching movement. Breathe in as you raise the arms, and exhale as they drop down. Repeat a few times.

2 Inhale and circle the arms out and up. Bring your hands above your head, palms facing. Breathing out, lower the arms to throat level: bend the elbows and turn the palms down. Move the hands down the center of the body, past the abdomen and out to the sides. Repeat.

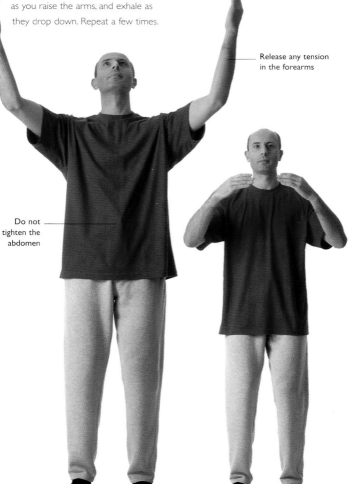

Release any tension in the forearms

Do not tighten the abdomen

Energy Work

After warming up, you may like to do some simple exercises to build energy in the body. The exercises given here should help you to establish a connection with the three main energy centers in the body. They may also help you to become familiar with the subtle movement of energy through the body.

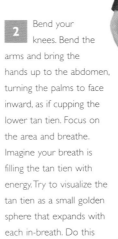

1 Stand erect, with your feet shoulder-width apart and parallel to each other. Gently rock from side to side, and front and back until your weight is equally balanced between your feet. Let your arms hang down by your sides, a little distance from your body. Relax the fingers, keeping them a little apart from each other. Look straight ahead.

2 Bend your knees. Bend the arms and bring the hands up to the abdomen, turning the palms to face inward, as if cupping the lower tan tien. Focus on the area and breathe. Imagine your breath is filling the tan tien with energy. Try to visualize the tan tien as a small golden sphere that expands with each in-breath. Do this for a minute or two.

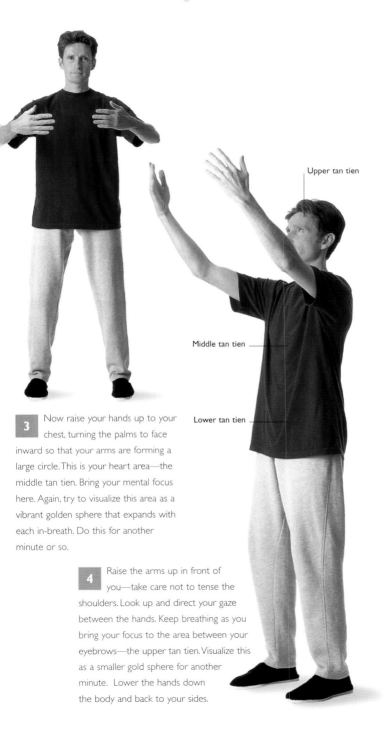

Upper tan tien

Middle tan tien

Lower tan tien

3 Now raise your hands up to your chest, turning the palms to face inward so that your arms are forming a large circle. This is your heart area—the middle tan tien. Bring your mental focus here. Again, try to visualize this area as a vibrant golden sphere that expands with each in-breath. Do this for another minute or so.

4 Raise the arms up in front of you—take care not to tense the shoulders. Look up and direct your gaze between the hands. Keep breathing as you bring your focus to the area between your eyebrows—the upper tan tien. Visualize this as a smaller gold sphere for another minute. Lower the hands down the body and back to your sides.

Energy Work

These postures, used in chi kung, help to release energy from the lower tan tien into the rest of the body. Some people may experience this as a sensation of warmth spreading outward from the belly; others may notice a feeling of release or relaxation. Occasionally people feel shaky or achy—this is said to be caused by blocked chi. Try to relax the area, and stop and rest if you feel dizzy.

MOTHER POSTURE

Stand in tai chi posture. Raise the arms and bend the elbows so that your arms form a circle in front of your body, with your hands at throat level. Keep the fingers relaxed and slightly apart. Hold the pose for 1–3 minutes, and breathe deeply. Be aware of tension creeping in: keep relaxing the belly and shoulders. This pose helps to direct chi all over the body.

FATHER POSTURE

Now, turn your hands so that the palms face outward. Hold the posture for 1–3 minutes, breathing into the abdomen and relaxing the belly and shoulders. Keep the fingers relaxed but not touching, and direct your gaze straight ahead. This posture is said to direct chi into the upper back, neck, and shoulders.

DAUGHTER POSTURE

Now lower the hands so that they are
pointing downward and slightly
inward. They should rest just
above your upper abdomen.
Keep the forearms straight,
as if letting water run down
them and drip into the ground.
Hold the pose for 1–3 minutes. This
sends chi into the elbows and forearms.

SON POSTURE

This pose directs chi into the wrists and hands.
Bring the hands down, palms facing each other
as if holding a ball. Keep the hands relaxed
and pointing slightly down. Keep some space
under the arms—do not let them touch the
body. Hold the pose for 1–3 minutes,
breathing deeply and noticing any feelings of
heat or tingling between the hands. End with
the Storing Energy pose on page 58.

Storing Energy

The energy exercises described in the previous pages serve to move chi around the body. It is important that you bring the chi back to the lower tan tien afterward. This simple exercise serves to store the energy so that it can be used in the tai chi form. You may notice that you feel stronger and more centered afterward.

Your mind is focused
on the lower tan tien

Chest is relaxed

STORING THE CHI

Place one hand on top of the other as you rest them on the lower abdomen, just below the navel. Focus your mind on the lower tan tien as you breathe naturally and quietly. This is said to direct the chi into the body's main energy store. Keep the belly and shoulders relaxed and close your eyes to help you to focus. Breathe for a minute or until you feel relaxed.

Hands rest gently
on the lower tan
tien, where energy
is stored

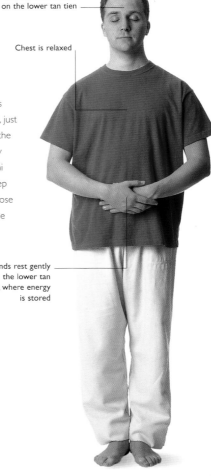

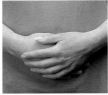

■ *Traditionally, women place the left hand over the right, while men place the right hand over the left.*

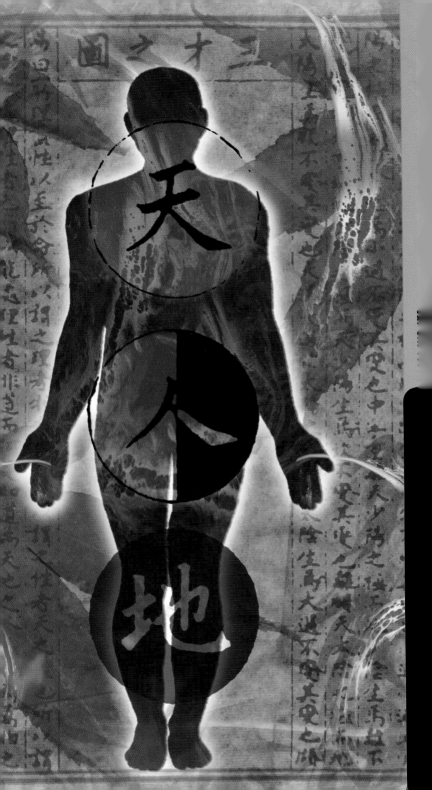

The Tai Chi Form

This is the traditional short form, which was devised by tai chi master Cheng Man-ching in the 1930s. Try to set aside ten minutes every day for your practice. Over time the intricate movements of the form will become second nature to you.

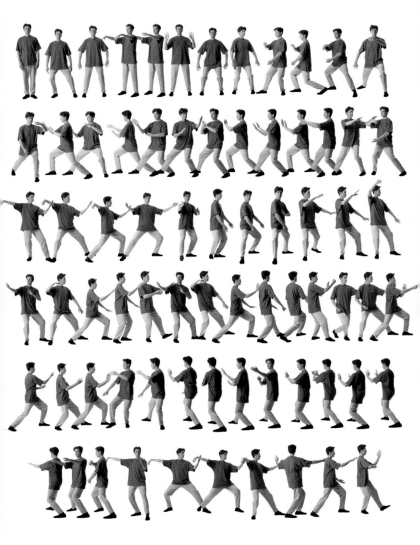

Points to Remember

There are four main points to remember when you are learning and practicing tai chi. First, and most importantly, relax. Release physical tension by warming up, and maintain good, relaxed posture throughout your practice. Relax the mind, too—quieten your thoughts by standing still and simply breathing for a few moments before you start.

Second, do not rush through the form. Take the time to learn the sequences properly, and keep your movements slow and controlled at all times. Third, keep the flow. Do not go so slowly that you lose interest and become frustrated. Let your movements come from the center of your body so that they are smooth and light.

Finally, develop precision in the practice. Although the tai chi is flowing and graceful, it involves precise movements that have been worked out over many years so that they benefit the body in particular ways. Use the final pose of each sequence to check your posture and alignment is correct. Always sink into the pose so that you experience it fully before gliding into the next sequence.

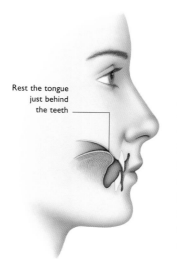

Rest the tongue just behind the teeth

DIRECTING THE CHI

Tai chi exercises are intended to move chi around the body. Your posture is very important—if it is tense or distorted, the flow of chi will be blocked. Your mind and breath also encourage the circulation of chi through the body. Remain mentally alert throughout the practice, and stay aware of your tan tien. Ideally, breathe into the lower abdomen but if you find this hard, simply breathe naturally— the most important thing is that you do not force or hold the breath. Place the tip of your tongue on the roof of your mouth, just behind the top teeth—this is said to help the flow of chi and also encourages relaxation and focus.

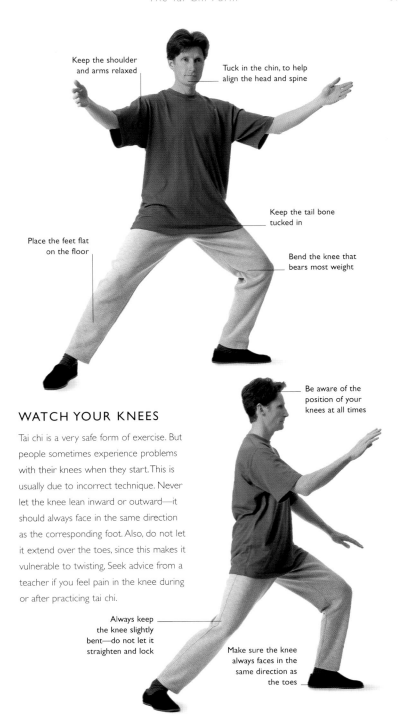

Keep the shoulder and arms relaxed

Tuck in the chin, to help align the head and spine

Keep the tail bone tucked in

Place the feet flat on the floor

Bend the knee that bears most weight

Be aware of the position of your knees at all times

WATCH YOUR KNEES

Tai chi is a very safe form of exercise. But people sometimes experience problems with their knees when they start. This is usually due to incorrect technique. Never let the knee lean inward or outward—it should always face in the same direction as the corresponding foot. Also, do not let it extend over the toes, since this makes it vulnerable to twisting, Seek advice from a teacher if you feel pain in the knee during or after practicing tai chi.

Always keep the knee slightly bent—do not let it straighten and lock

Make sure the knee always faces in the same direction as the toes

Opening

You should always do tai chi in a relaxed frame of mind. Spend a few moments standing quietly before you begin, breathing deeply and letting tension drain from your body. Then, slowly move into the opening stance. As you do so, imagine your head is suspended from a thread that is attached to the crown, as if you were a puppet on a string. With practice, this should lead to a sense of lightness and release, which is the ideal state for the practice of tai chi.

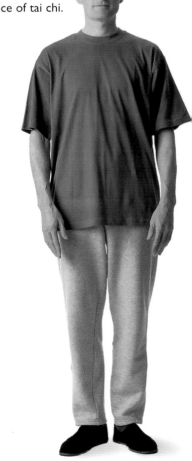

1 Stand upright, facing forward. Tuck in your chin and your tail bone. Place your heels so they are close together but not touching, with your toes pointing outward. Your weight should be equally balanced between the two feet. Relax your shoulders and let your arms hang down, keeping a space between them and your body. Your fingers, too, should be slightly apart rather than touching. Do not lock the elbows or knees—they should be bent.

CENTER POINT

In tai chi all movements emanate from the point called the tan tien. This is the energy center which lies just below and behind your navel. Stay aware of this area as you practice, and let it act as a guide to your movements.

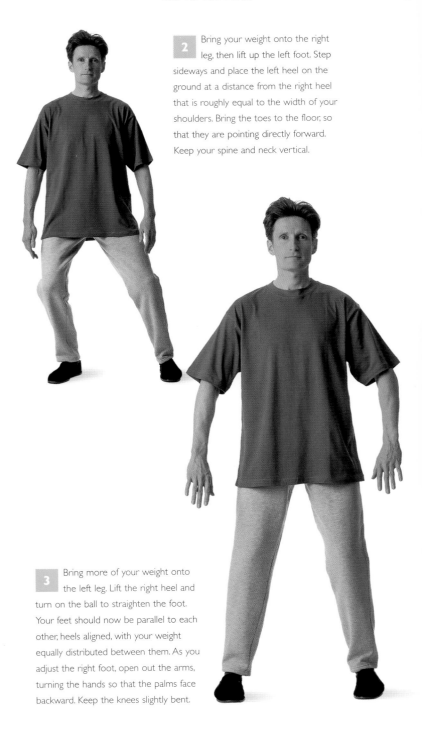

2 Bring your weight onto the right leg, then lift up the left foot. Step sideways and place the left heel on the ground at a distance from the right heel that is roughly equal to the width of your shoulders. Bring the toes to the floor, so that they are pointing directly forward. Keep your spine and neck vertical.

3 Bring more of your weight onto the left leg. Lift the right heel and turn on the ball to straighten the foot. Your feet should now be parallel to each other, heels aligned, with your weight equally distributed between them. As you adjust the right foot, open out the arms, turning the hands so that the palms face backward. Keep the knees slightly bent.

Beginning

In this first sequence, the arms are raised in a seemingly effortless movement. Let them rise upward, as though they are being lifted by threads at the wrists and elbows. Keep the shoulders relaxed.

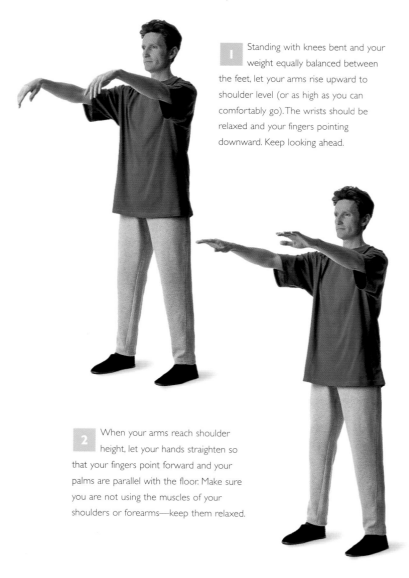

1 Standing with knees bent and your weight equally balanced between the feet, let your arms rise upward to shoulder level (or as high as you can comfortably go). The wrists should be relaxed and your fingers pointing downward. Keep looking ahead.

2 When your arms reach shoulder height, let your hands straighten so that your fingers point forward and your palms are parallel with the floor. Make sure you are not using the muscles of your shoulders or forearms—keep them relaxed.

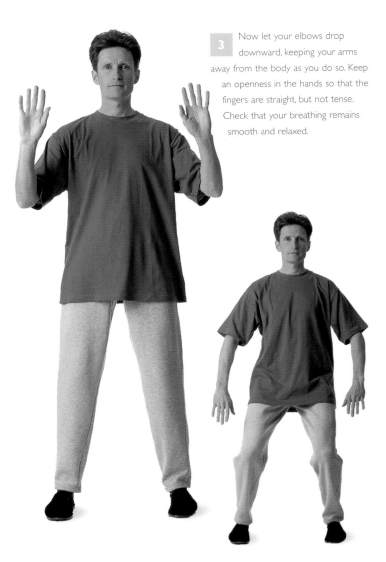

3 Now let your elbows drop downward, keeping your arms away from the body as you do so. Keep an openness in the hands so that the fingers are straight, but not tense. Check that your breathing remains smooth and relaxed.

4 Keeping the space between your arms and your body, let your forearms drop down. Let your weight sink down into the ground, while still retaining the feeling that your head is suspended from a thread. Your weight should remain equally balanced between your two feet.

Opening

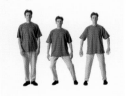

Turn to the Right

This sequence introduces a movement known as holding the ball, which is used many times in the form. Your hands are held in front of the body, palms facing each other as if there were a large ball between them. Try to imagine you are holding a ball of energy; this will help you to synchronize the movement of your arms with the turns of your waist into one flowing sequence.

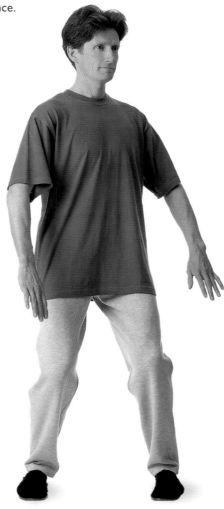

1 Sink most of your weight into the left leg, bending the left knee and starting to straighten the right leg as you do so. Slowly turn the body to the left, while keeping your feet in their position. Your arms should still be by your sides, but not touching them.

PROTECTING THE KNEES

Tai chi can be hard on your knees if done incorrectly. As you bring more weight into a leg, bend the knee well. Let the other leg straighten, but always keep a slight bend in the knee.

2 Now raise the right toes. Turn your foot on its heel to the right. At the same time, turn your upper body in the same direction. As you turn, raise the right arm. Turn the palm down as though it is resting on top of a ball. The left palm turns to face upward, as if supporting the base. Place the right foot flat on the floor, and start to bring your weight onto the right leg.

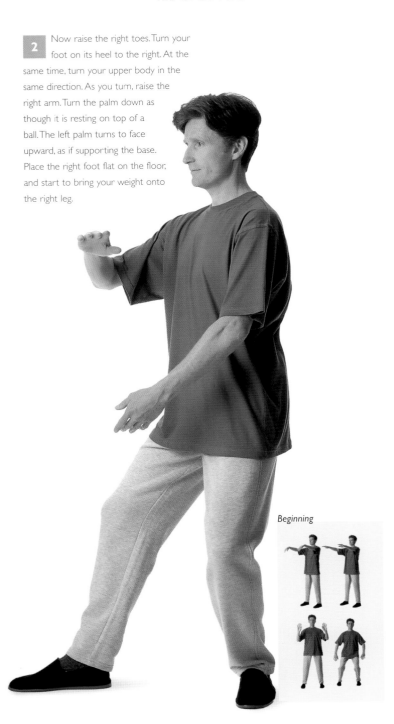

Beginning

Ward Off Left

This is a strong stance in which you are firmly rooted in the ground. Make sure that you keep sinking your weight downward. Your knees should be in line with the toes, not bending inward or outward.

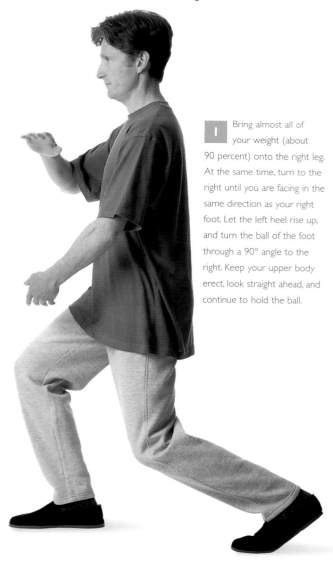

1 Bring almost all of your weight (about 90 percent) onto the right leg. At the same time, turn to the right until you are facing in the same direction as your right foot. Let the left heel rise up, and turn the ball of the foot through a 90° angle to the right. Keep your upper body erect, look straight ahead, and continue to hold the ball.

2 Bringing all your weight onto the right leg, step the left foot out to your left. Place the heel down first, then roll the toes down onto the floor. The left foot should be at right angles to the right, at a distance that is equal to one and a half times the width of your shoulders. Make sure that the left knee points in the same direction as the left toes.

3 Move 70 percent of your weight onto the left leg. Raise your left arm in front of the chest, palm facing you. Drop the right arm to your side, palm facing back. The hands pass smoothly over each other in this action. At the same time, turn your waist to the left to face forward. Lift your right toes and turn them toward the front. This is the bow and arrow stance.

Turn to the Right

Ward Off Right

This movement follows on in a seamless flow from Ward Off Left. Breathe steadily and smoothly as you move, keeping your head and spine in alignment, chin and tail bone tucked in.

1 Bring most of your weight onto the left leg and raise the right heel. Turn your waist slightly to the left. At the same time, move the left hand to face downward. Move the right arm forward and turn the palm upward to hold the ball.

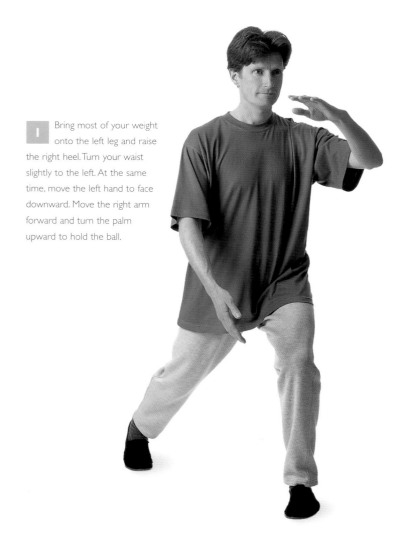

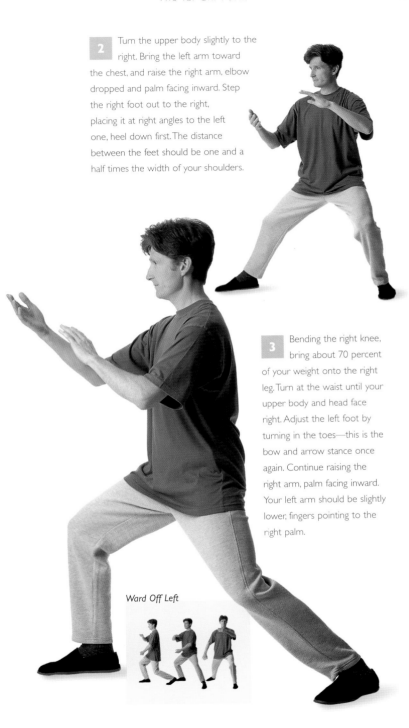

2 Turn the upper body slightly to the right. Bring the left arm toward the chest, and raise the right arm, elbow dropped and palm facing inward. Step the right foot out to the right, placing it at right angles to the left one, heel down first. The distance between the feet should be one and a half times the width of your shoulders.

3 Bending the right knee, bring about 70 percent of your weight onto the right leg. Turn at the waist until your upper body and head face right. Adjust the left foot by turning in the toes—this is the bow and arrow stance once again. Continue raising the right arm, palm facing inward. Your left arm should be slightly lower, fingers pointing to the right palm.

Ward Off Left

Rollback

This is a pose in which energy is drawn inward, to prepare for the outward movements of Press and Push that follow. Try not to stop at any point—advanced practitioners in tai chi do all the movements in this sequence during one inward breath. Keep your body soft—in particular try to relax the hips so that the waist can move freely.

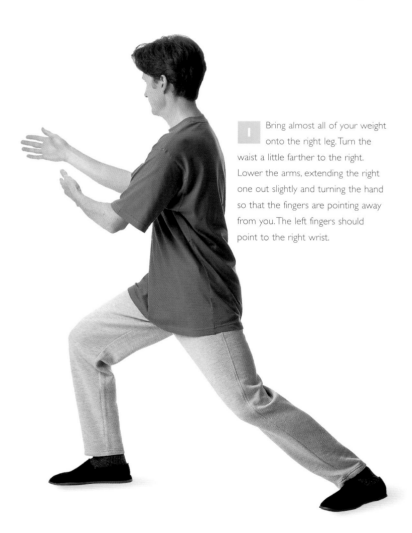

1 Bring almost all of your weight onto the right leg. Turn the waist a little farther to the right. Lower the arms, extending the right one out slightly and turning the hand so that the fingers are pointing away from you. The left fingers should point to the right wrist.

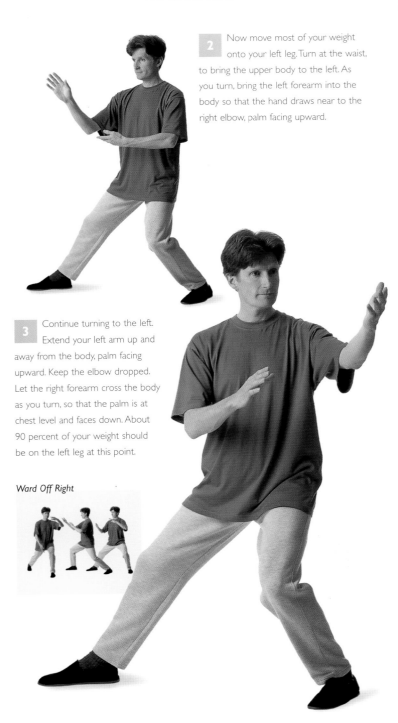

2 Now move most of your weight onto your left leg. Turn at the waist, to bring the upper body to the left. As you turn, bring the left forearm into the body so that the hand draws near to the right elbow, palm facing upward.

3 Continue turning to the left. Extend your left arm up and away from the body, palm facing upward. Keep the elbow dropped. Let the right forearm cross the body as you turn, so that the palm is at chest level and faces down. About 90 percent of your weight should be on the left leg at this point.

Ward Off Right

Press

After drawing energy into the body through the Rollback sequence, you now send it outward. As you press forward, make sure that you maintain a strong stance and keep your feet firmly rooted into the ground. Watch that your shoulders do not rise up; they should remain relaxed at all times during the form.

1 Keep your feet in the same position as in Rollback. Bring your weight onto the right leg as you turn the waist to the right. Raise the right forearm, palm facing toward you. At the same time, bring the left arm right up and rest the left palm gently on the right one.

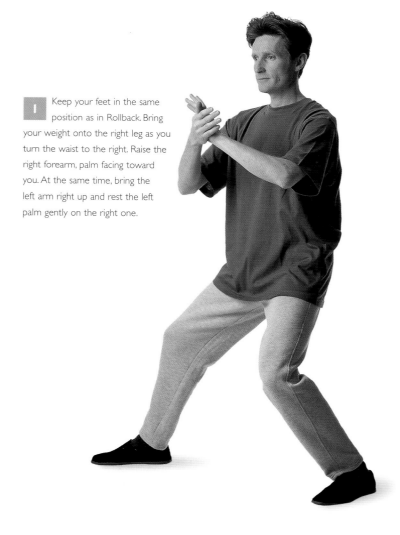

2 Continue the turn until you are facing right, but do not move your feet out of the bow and arrow stance. Increase the weight on your right leg and push forward with the upper body and arms. Do not raise the back heel off the ground. Keep the spine and head upright. About 70 percent of your weight should be on the right leg at this point.

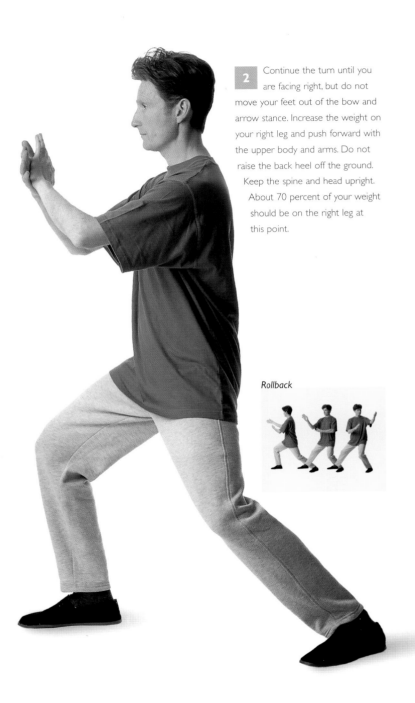

Rollback

Push

This is an energizing final pose which can be practiced on its own to boost energy and increase concentration levels. As with the previous movement, be sure to keep your feet flat on the ground as you push.

1 Slowly separate out your hands until they are both at shoulder height with your palms facing downward. Keep the fingers slightly bent. Bring most of your body weight onto the left leg. Bend the left knee and keep the right knee soft. Relax in the hips.

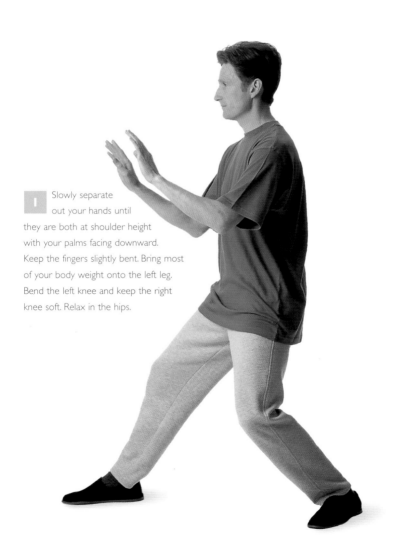

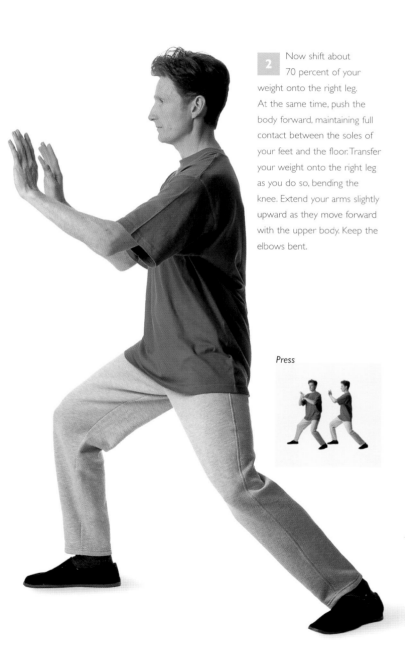

2 Now shift about 70 percent of your weight onto the right leg. At the same time, push the body forward, maintaining full contact between the soles of your feet and the floor. Transfer your weight onto the right leg as you do so, bending the knee. Extend your arms slightly upward as they move forward with the upper body. Keep the elbows bent.

Press

Turning the Body

This turn leads into Single Whip, an intricate sequence that requires great concentration and control. Take the time to become familiar with all the different moves, so that you can perform them in a graceful way without having to keep stopping and starting. Single Whip appears five times in the form.

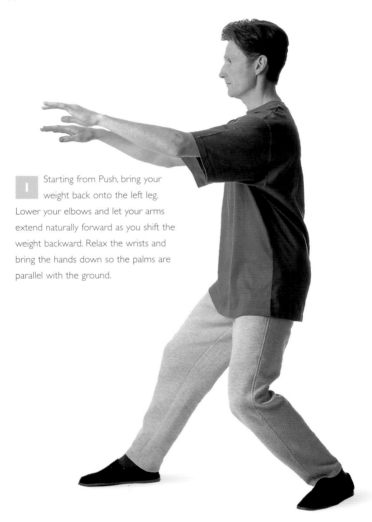

1 Starting from Push, bring your weight back onto the left leg. Lower your elbows and let your arms extend naturally forward as you shift the weight backward. Relax the wrists and bring the hands down so the palms are parallel with the ground.

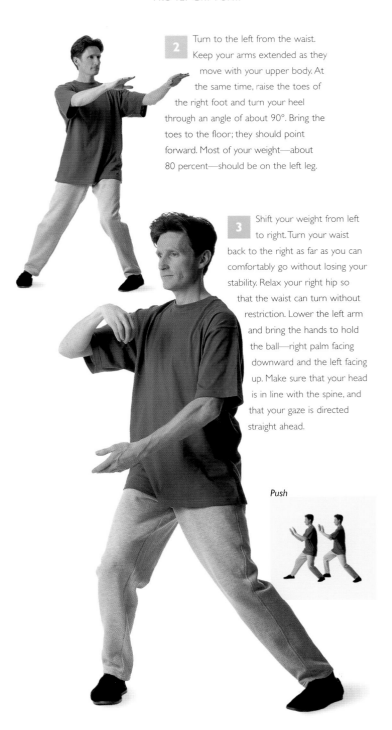

2 Turn to the left from the waist. Keep your arms extended as they move with your upper body. At the same time, raise the toes of the right foot and turn your heel through an angle of about 90°. Bring the toes to the floor; they should point forward. Most of your weight—about 80 percent—should be on the left leg.

3 Shift your weight from left to right. Turn your waist back to the right as far as you can comfortably go without losing your stability. Relax your right hip so that the waist can turn without restriction. Lower the left arm and bring the hands to hold the ball—right palm facing downward and the left facing up. Make sure that your head is in line with the spine, and that your gaze is directed straight ahead.

Push

Single Whip

You now move into Single Whip. In the final position, you bring your right hand into a loose hook or beak shape. Be sure to keep shoulder, elbow, and wrist relaxed as you settle into the pose.

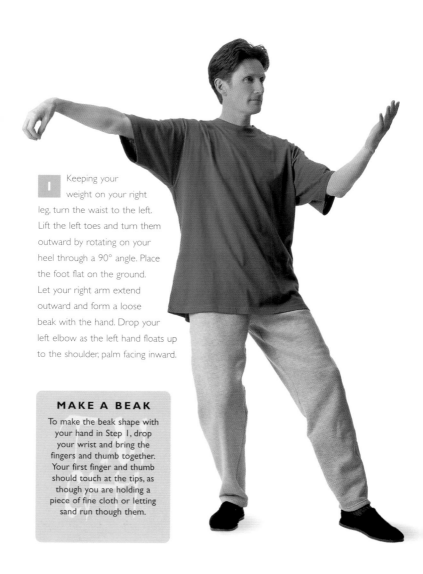

I Keeping your weight on your right leg, turn the waist to the left. Lift the left toes and turn them outward by rotating on your heel through a 90° angle. Place the foot flat on the ground. Let your right arm extend outward and form a loose beak with the hand. Drop your left elbow as the left hand floats up to the shoulder, palm facing inward.

MAKE A BEAK

To make the beak shape with your hand in Step 1, drop your wrist and bring the fingers and thumb together. Your first finger and thumb should touch at the tips, as though you are holding a piece of fine cloth or letting sand run though them.

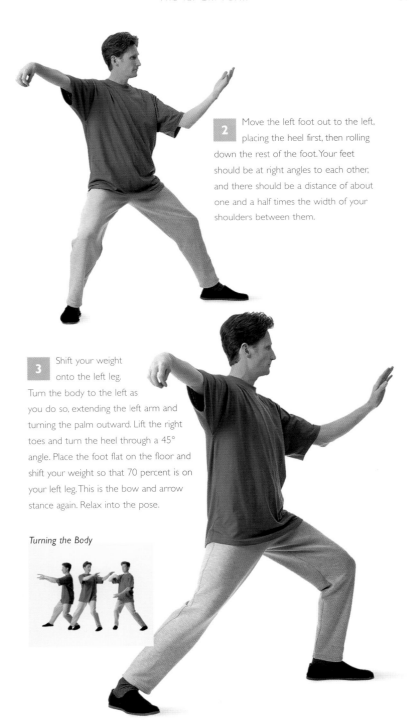

2 Move the left foot out to the left, placing the heel first, then rolling down the rest of the foot. Your feet should be at right angles to each other, and there should be a distance of about one and a half times the width of your shoulders between them.

3 Shift your weight onto the left leg. Turn the body to the left as you do so, extending the left arm and turning the palm outward. Lift the right toes and turn the heel through a 45° angle. Place the foot flat on the floor and shift your weight so that 70 percent is on your left leg. This is the bow and arrow stance again. Relax into the pose.

Turning the Body

Lifting Hands

In this sequence, you open the arms wide, as if you are gathering energy from the atmosphere and bringing it toward the body. It has a rejuvenating effect after the focused effort of Single Whip. Lifting Hands is a good sequence to practice on its own, as it helps to strengthen the legs and improve your stability and grounding.

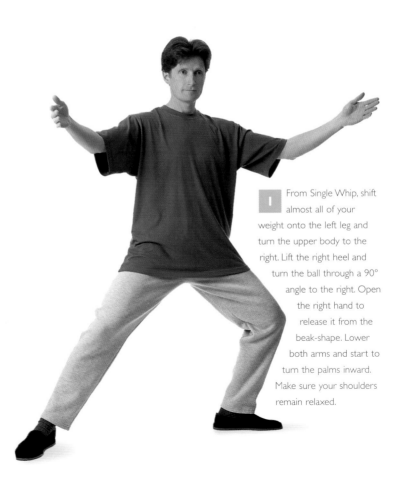

1 From Single Whip, shift almost all of your weight onto the left leg and turn the upper body to the right. Lift the right heel and turn the ball through a 90° angle to the right. Open the right hand to release it from the beak-shape. Lower both arms and start to turn the palms inward. Make sure your shoulders remain relaxed.

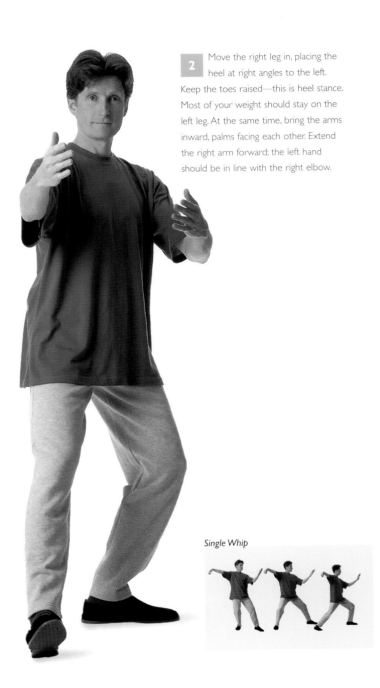

2 Move the right leg in, placing the heel at right angles to the left. Keep the toes raised—this is heel stance. Most of your weight should stay on the left leg. At the same time, bring the arms inward, palms facing each other. Extend the right arm forward; the left hand should be in line with the right elbow.

Single Whip

Shoulder Stroke

In this powerful sequence, your weight shifts from left to right. Make sure that the supporting foot remains firmly rooted in the ground, and that you do not push the knee out of alignment as you turn.

1 Bring all your weight onto the left leg. Step the right foot toward the left one, placing the toes next to the left heel. Leave the right heel raised up. At the same time, turn the waist to the left and lower your arms in front of the body. The palms should be facing each other.

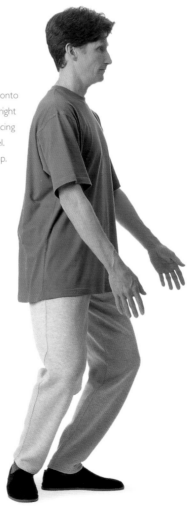

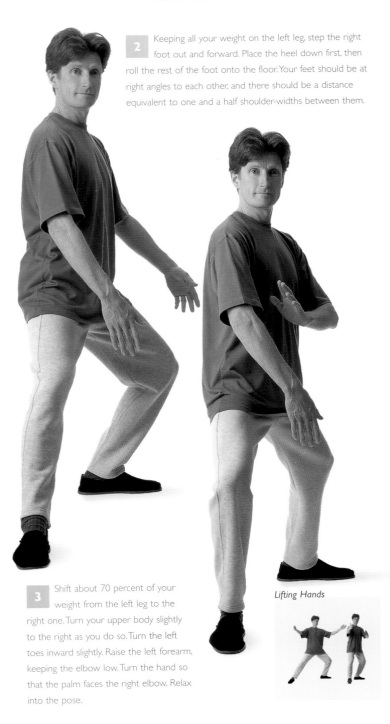

2 Keeping all your weight on the left leg, step the right foot out and forward. Place the heel down first, then roll the rest of the foot onto the floor. Your feet should be at right angles to each other, and there should be a distance equivalent to one and a half shoulder-widths between them.

3 Shift about 70 percent of your weight from the left leg to the right one. Turn your upper body slightly to the right as you do so. Turn the left toes inward slightly. Raise the left forearm, keeping the elbow low. Turn the hand so that the palm faces the right elbow. Relax into the pose.

Lifting Hands

White Crane Spreads Its Wings

This is a beautiful movement, based on the graceful action of a crane spreading its wings. The front of the body is expansive and open. The right arm extends up and the left one drops downward, forming a connection with both the earth and the sky.

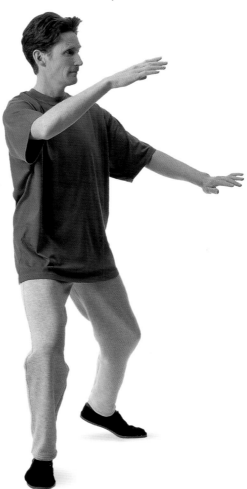

1 Bring all of your weight onto the right leg. Raise the right arm, bending the elbow. Turn your waist slightly to the left, and extend the left arm out and down. Raise your left heel off the floor.

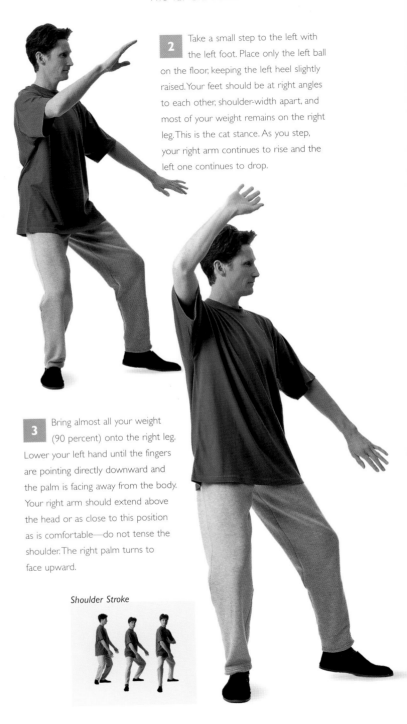

2 Take a small step to the left with the left foot. Place only the left ball on the floor, keeping the left heel slightly raised. Your feet should be at right angles to each other, shoulder-width apart, and most of your weight remains on the right leg. This is the cat stance. As you step, your right arm continues to rise and the left one continues to drop.

3 Bring almost all your weight (90 percent) onto the right leg. Lower your left hand until the fingers are pointing directly downward and the palm is facing away from the body. Your right arm should extend above the head or as close to this position as is comfortable—do not tense the shoulder. The right palm turns to face upward.

Shoulder Stroke

Brush Left Knee and Push

This fluid sequence appears twice in the form. The right leg and left arm work together, as do the left leg and right arm. As you become more practiced at tai chi, you will be able to create a smooth coordination of movement between the different sides of the body.

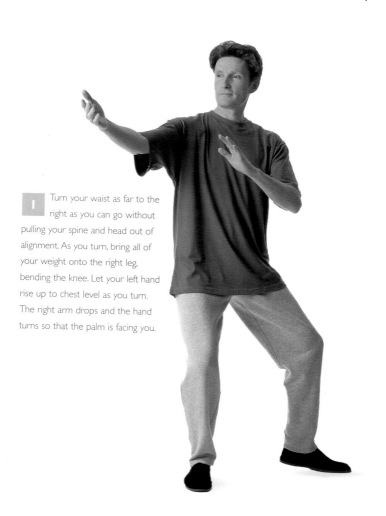

1 Turn your waist as far to the right as you can go without pulling your spine and head out of alignment. As you turn, bring all of your weight onto the right leg, bending the knee. Let your left hand rise up to chest level as you turn. The right arm drops and the hand turns so that the palm is facing you.

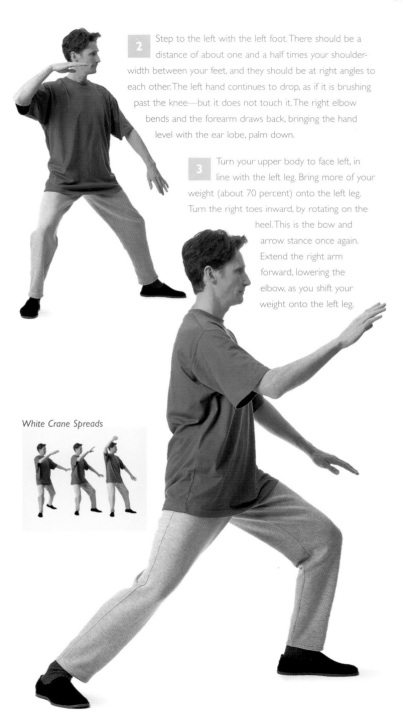

2 Step to the left with the left foot. There should be a distance of about one and a half times your shoulder-width between your feet, and they should be at right angles to each other. The left hand continues to drop, as if it is brushing past the knee—but it does not touch it. The right elbow bends and the forearm draws back, bringing the hand level with the ear lobe, palm down.

3 Turn your upper body to face left, in line with the left leg. Bring more of your weight (about 70 percent) onto the left leg. Turn the right toes inward, by rotating on the heel. This is the bow and arrow stance once again. Extend the right arm forward, lowering the elbow, as you shift your weight onto the left leg.

White Crane Spreads

Play the Lute

In this sequence, you position the hands as if you are about to strum the strings of a lute or guitar. Concentrate on your timing, and synchronize the movements into one harmonious whole. As you relax into the final pose, try to feel energy vibrating between your hands.

I Bring all your weight into the left leg. Move the right foot in, placing it just behind the left foot and at a 45° angle to it. Place the toes down first, then roll the foot onto the floor.

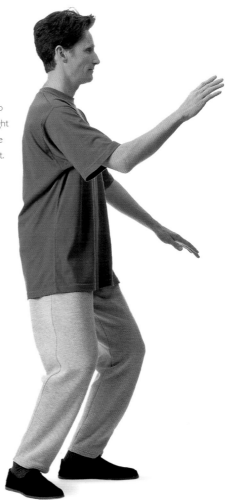

2 Shift all your weight onto the right leg and turn your upper body to the right. Raise the left arm and lower the right to bring them both to chest level. Turn the palms inward. Move the left foot forward and to the left, so the feet are shoulder-width apart. Keep the toes raised—this is heel stance.

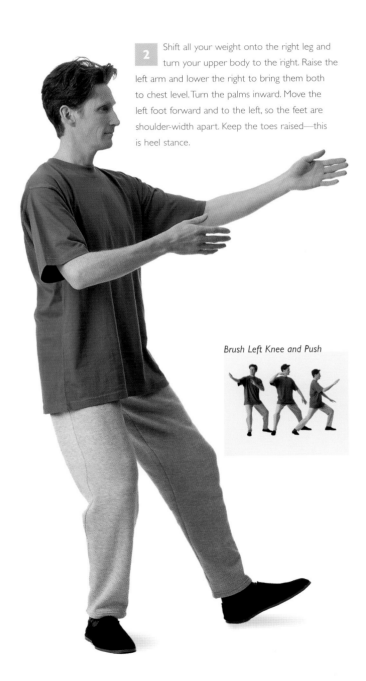

Brush Left Knee and Push

Brush Left
Knee and Push

This is the second time that Brush Left Knee appears in the form. The movement is the same, but this time you begin from the heel stance of Play the Lute rather than the toe stance of White Crane. Again, the right leg works with the left arm and vice versa. Concentrate on creating a smooth, synchronized movement.

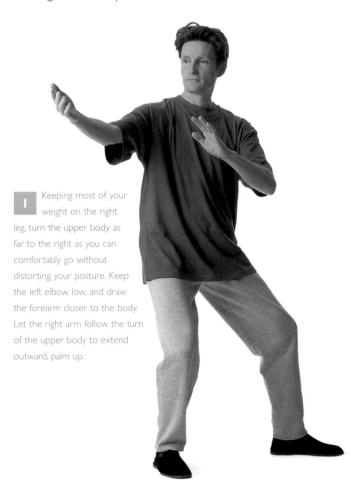

1 Keeping most of your weight on the right leg, turn the upper body as far to the right as you can comfortably go without distorting your posture. Keep the left elbow low, and draw the forearm closer to the body. Let the right arm follow the turn of the upper body to extend outward, palm up.

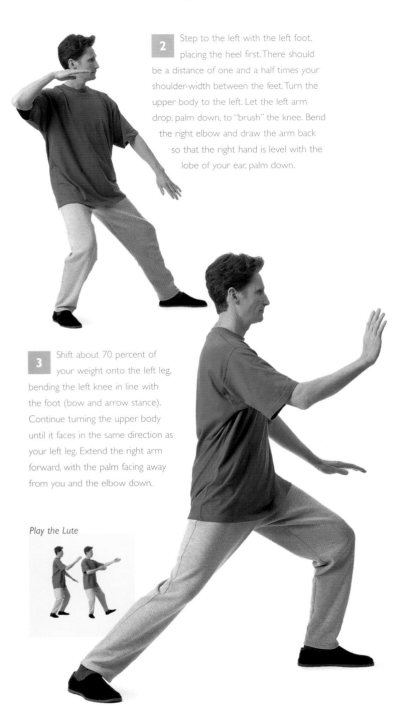

2 Step to the left with the left foot, placing the heel first. There should be a distance of one and a half times your shoulder-width between the feet. Turn the upper body to the left. Let the left arm drop, palm down, to "brush" the knee. Bend the right elbow and draw the arm back so that the right hand is level with the lobe of your ear, palm down.

3 Shift about 70 percent of your weight onto the left leg, bending the left knee in line with the foot (bow and arrow stance). Continue turning the upper body until it faces in the same direction as your left leg. Extend the right arm forward, with the palm facing away from you and the elbow down.

Play the Lute

Step Forward and Deflect

This is the start of an empowering sequence that builds strength and self-confidence. It also requires good balance. Try to let your actions be guided from the energy center (tan tien) in the lower abdomen. Keep your arms relaxed so that they can follow the waist as it turns in one flowing movement.

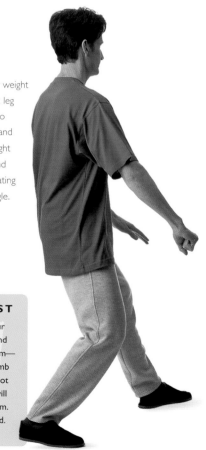

1 Drop most of your weight back onto the right leg and turn the upper body to the left. Lower both arms and make a soft fist with the right hand. Raise the left toes and turn them outward by rotating the heel through a 45° angle. Place the foot down flat.

MAKING A FIST

To form a fist, curl your fingers into the hand and bend the thumb over them— do not enclose the thumb within the fingers. Do not clench the fist as this will create tension in the arm. Keep it firm but relaxed.

2 Shift all your weight onto the left leg, and let the right heel rise up. Continue turning the upper body to the left until you are facing in the same direction as the left foot. Remember to keep the knees aligned with the feet.

3 Step your right foot forward, placing the heel down first and in line with the arch of the left foot. There should be a 90° angle between the feet. As you step, turn the waist to the right. Let your arms rise, elbows down. Your left palm should face the right wrist.

Brush Left Knee and Push

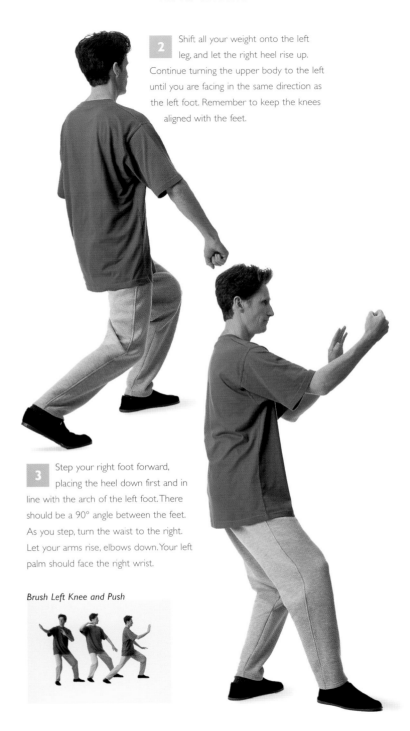

Parry and Punch

These steps complete the sequence started with **Step Forward and Deflect**. Mind the temptation to hurry when you get to the final punch—keep your movements controlled and slow.

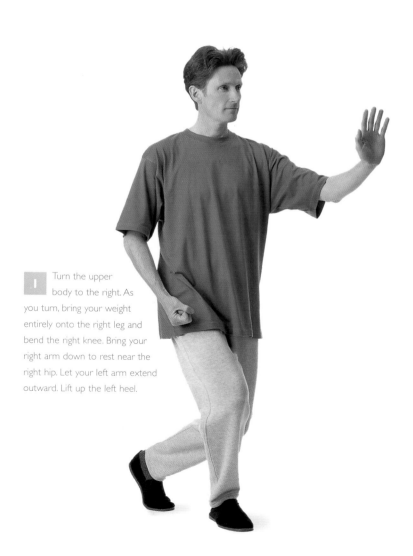

1 Turn the upper body to the right. As you turn, bring your weight entirely onto the right leg and bend the right knee. Bring your right arm down to rest near the right hip. Let your left arm extend outward. Lift up the left heel.

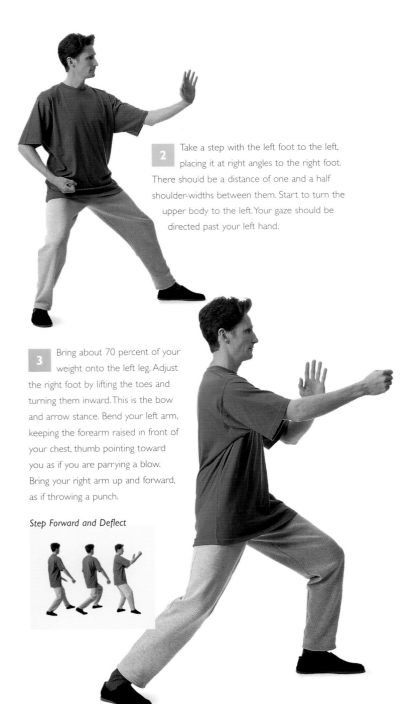

2 Take a step with the left foot to the left, placing it at right angles to the right foot. There should be a distance of one and a half shoulder-widths between them. Start to turn the upper body to the left. Your gaze should be directed past your left hand.

3 Bring about 70 percent of your weight onto the left leg. Adjust the right foot by lifting the toes and turning them inward. This is the bow and arrow stance. Bend your left arm, keeping the forearm raised in front of your chest, thumb pointing toward you as if you are parrying a blow. Bring your right arm up and forward, as if throwing a punch.

Step Forward and Deflect

Withdraw and Push

This is a relaxing sequence, which helps to release the energy built up in the Punch. You first draw back and then push forward, moving with the upper body without changing the position of the feet. The arm movements help to loosen and mobilize the wrists and elbows. Keep your head and spine in alignment—tuck in the chin and tail bone.

I Turn the upper body to the left. Release the right hand from its fist, and turn the palm to face upward. Drop the left forearm and turn the wrist so that the hand is close to the right elbow, palm facing upward. Remember to keep some space between the arms and the sides of your body.

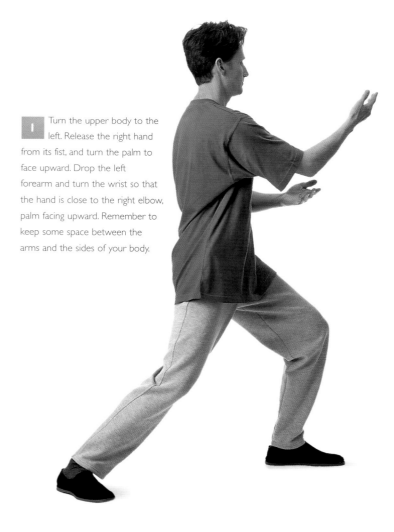

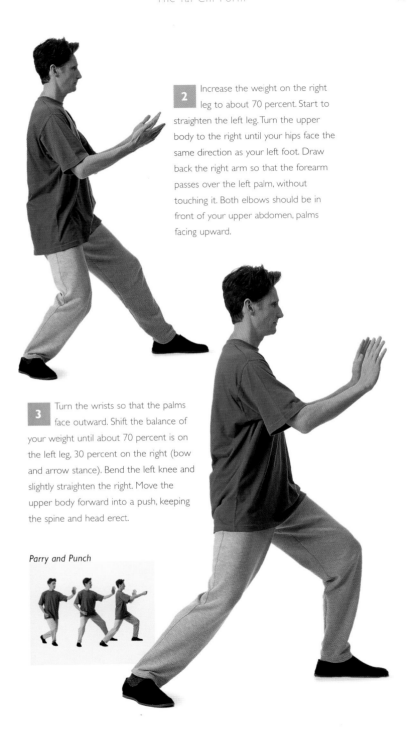

2 Increase the weight on the right leg to about 70 percent. Start to straighten the left leg. Turn the upper body to the right until your hips face the same direction as your left foot. Draw back the right arm so that the forearm passes over the left palm, without touching it. Both elbows should be in front of your upper abdomen, palms facing upward.

3 Turn the wrists so that the palms face outward. Shift the balance of your weight until about 70 percent is on the left leg, 30 percent on the right (bow and arrow stance). Bend the left knee and slightly straighten the right. Move the upper body forward into a push, keeping the spine and head erect.

Parry and Punch

Crossing Hands

In this sequence, you turn to face forward once again. As in Lifting Hands, it offers an opportunity to gather energy from the atmosphere and bring it toward the body. You can practice the final posture on its own, to build strength in the back and legs.

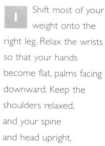 Shift most of your weight onto the right leg. Relax the wrists so that your hands become flat, palms facing downward. Keep the shoulders relaxed, and your spine and head upright.

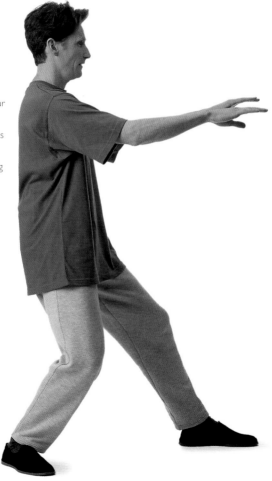

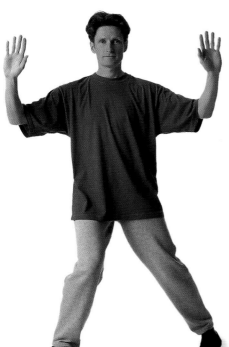

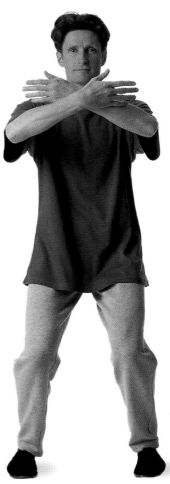

2 Turn your upper body to the right, so that you are facing forward again. As you turn, lift the toes of the left foot and rotate on the heel so that the foot is pointing forward. Let your arms open out as you turn. Both arms bend at the elbow and the palms turn outward. Make sure that you are maintaining a little space between your fingers.

3 Step with the right foot placing it parallel to the left. They should be shoulder-width apart. Drop the hands, then bring them up across the center of the body, crossing right wrist over left. The hands should be at throat level, with the palms facing inward. Shift your weight so about 60 percent of it is on the left leg.

Withdraw and Push

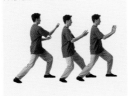

Embrace Tiger,
Return to Mountain

This sequence helps to loosen the hips. It requires you to take a long step, which can make keeping your balance difficult. Remember to ground yourself by bringing all your weight onto the left leg before you step. Check that you do not hold your breath at any stage—in tai chi, the breath like the movement forms one continuous flow.

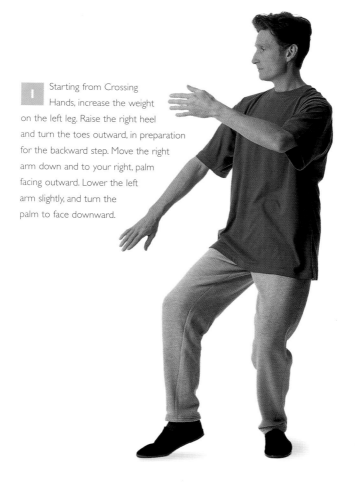

1 Starting from Crossing Hands, increase the weight on the left leg. Raise the right heel and turn the toes outward, in preparation for the backward step. Move the right arm down and to your right, palm facing outward. Lower the left arm slightly, and turn the palm to face downward.

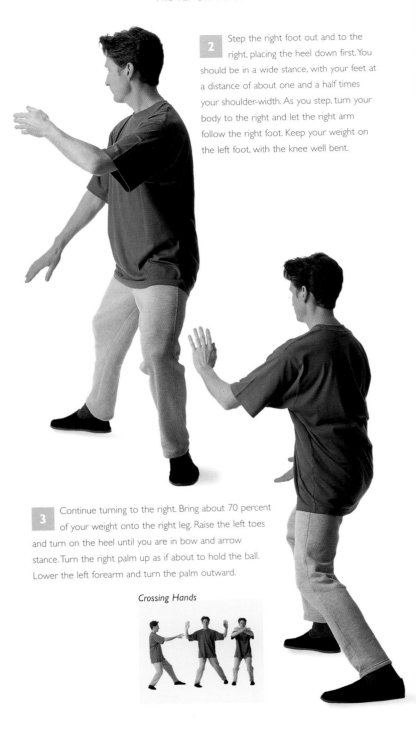

2 Step the right foot out and to the right, placing the heel down first. You should be in a wide stance, with your feet at a distance of about one and a half times your shoulder-width. As you step, turn your body to the right and let the right arm follow the right foot. Keep your weight on the left foot, with the knee well bent.

3 Continue turning to the right. Bring about 70 percent of your weight onto the right leg. Raise the left toes and turn on the heel until you are in bow and arrow stance. Turn the right palm up as if about to hold the ball. Lower the left forearm and turn the palm outward.

Crossing Hands

Rollback

Rollback is the start of a series of movements that have already appeared in the form, and are repeated several more times. Exactly the same movements are performed as before, but this time you step in a different direction—to the back and right.

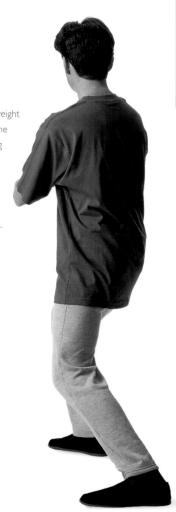

I Keeping most of your weight on the right leg, move the upper body to the right, turning from the waist and letting the tan tien (energy center in the lower abdomen) guide your movements. Lift your right hand and start to lower the left.

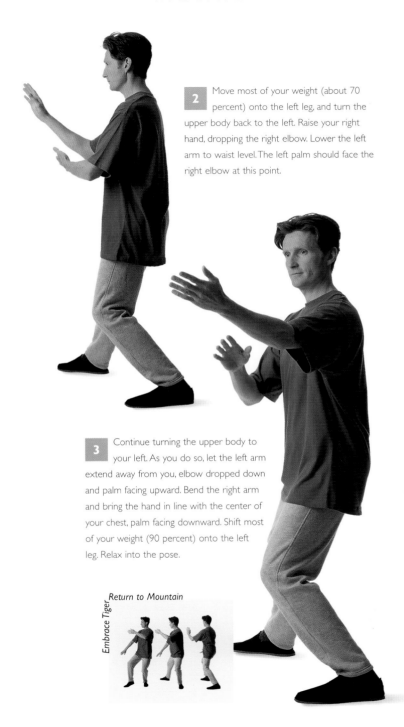

2 Move most of your weight (about 70 percent) onto the left leg, and turn the upper body back to the left. Raise your right hand, dropping the right elbow. Lower the left arm to waist level. The left palm should face the right elbow at this point.

3 Continue turning the upper body to your left. As you do so, let the left arm extend away from you, elbow dropped down and palm facing upward. Bend the right arm and bring the hand in line with the center of your chest, palm facing downward. Shift most of your weight (90 percent) onto the left leg. Relax into the pose.

Embrace Tiger   Return to Mountain

Press and Push

From the relaxing sequence of Rollback, you move into the outward movements of Press and Push. These serve to release energy from the body. Make sure that your posture remains upright but relaxed as you shift your weight from one leg to the other.

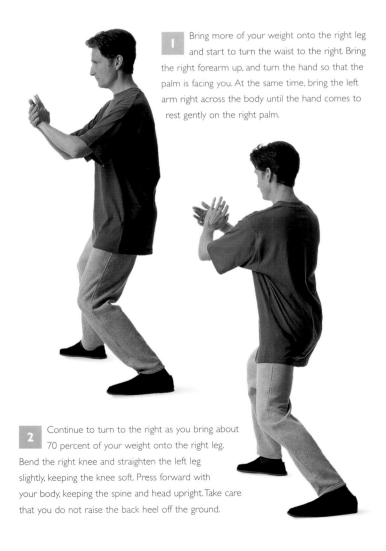

1 Bring more of your weight onto the right leg and start to turn the waist to the right. Bring the right forearm up, and turn the hand so that the palm is facing you. At the same time, bring the left arm right across the body until the hand comes to rest gently on the right palm.

2 Continue to turn to the right as you bring about 70 percent of your weight onto the right leg. Bend the right knee and straighten the left leg slightly, keeping the knee soft. Press forward with your body, keeping the spine and head upright. Take care that you do not raise the back heel off the ground.

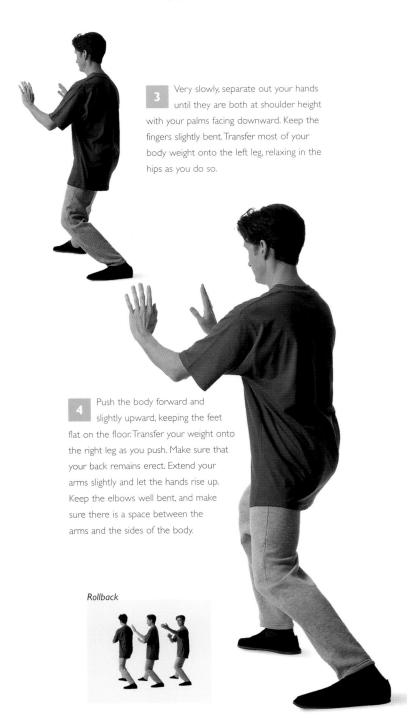

3 Very slowly, separate out your hands until they are both at shoulder height with your palms facing downward. Keep the fingers slightly bent. Transfer most of your body weight onto the left leg, relaxing in the hips as you do so.

4 Push the body forward and slightly upward, keeping the feet flat on the floor. Transfer your weight onto the right leg as you push. Make sure that your back remains erect. Extend your arms slightly and let the hands rise up. Keep the elbows well bent, and make sure there is a space between the arms and the sides of the body.

Rollback

Single Whip

Here, you turn to the left before moving into the Single Whip position. Take care to balance your weight correctly between your feet, and to keep your posture relaxed and stable. This will help you to glide through the intricate movements.

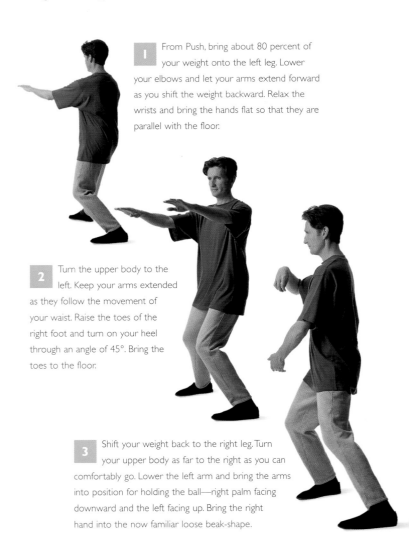

1 From Push, bring about 80 percent of your weight onto the left leg. Lower your elbows and let your arms extend forward as you shift the weight backward. Relax the wrists and bring the hands flat so that they are parallel with the floor.

2 Turn the upper body to the left. Keep your arms extended as they follow the movement of your waist. Raise the toes of the right foot and turn on your heel through an angle of 45°. Bring the toes to the floor.

3 Shift your weight back to the right leg. Turn your upper body as far to the right as you can comfortably go. Lower the left arm and bring the arms into position for holding the ball—right palm facing downward and the left facing up. Bring the right hand into the now familiar loose beak-shape.

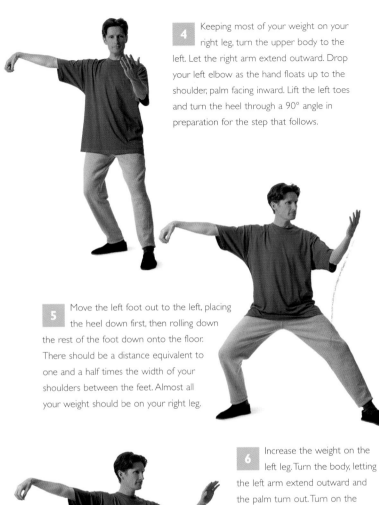

4 Keeping most of your weight on your right leg, turn the upper body to the left. Let the right arm extend outward. Drop your left elbow as the hand floats up to the shoulder, palm facing inward. Lift the left toes and turn the heel through a 90° angle in preparation for the step that follows.

5 Move the left foot out to the left, placing the heel down first, then rolling down the rest of the foot down onto the floor. There should be a distance equivalent to one and a half times the width of your shoulders between the feet. Almost all your weight should be on your right leg.

6 Increase the weight on the left leg. Turn the body, letting the left arm extend outward and the palm turn out. Turn on the right heel so that the toes point forward, in bow and arrow stance. Adjust your weight so that 70 percent of it is on the left leg.

Press and Push

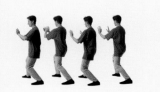

Punch under Elbow

This energizing sequence begins with expansive arm movements that help to release tension in the upper back. You step slowly forward, shifting your weight from one leg to the other in quick succession. The fist should be firm but loose, as though you are carrying a tiny bird. Make sure that your thumb folds over your fingers, not inside them.

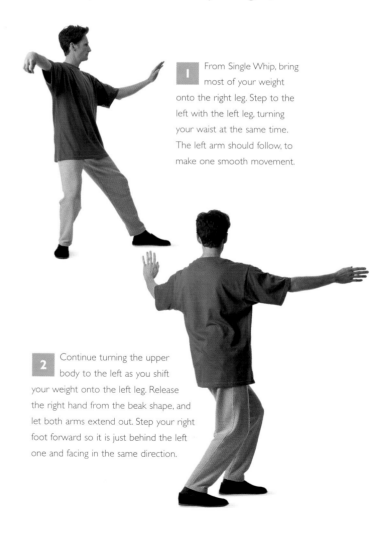

1 From Single Whip, bring most of your weight onto the right leg. Step to the left with the left leg, turning your waist at the same time. The left arm should follow, to make one smooth movement.

2 Continue turning the upper body to the left as you shift your weight onto the left leg. Release the right hand from the beak shape, and let both arms extend out. Step your right foot forward so it is just behind the left one and facing in the same direction.

3 Keeping most of your weight on the left leg, step back with the right foot, turning the toes outward slightly. Place the toes down first. At the same time, turn the upper body to the right. Lower the left arm, then start to bring it forward, palm facing upward as if you are scooping up water. At the same time, bend the right arm at the elbow, and turn the palm downward.

4 Shift all your weight onto the right leg. Raise the left toes, and move the left foot back. Keep the toes raised—this is heel stance. Raise the left arm in front of you, elbow dropped and fingers pointing up. Draw the right forearm across your chest, and bring the hand into a fist, facing the left elbow.

Single Whip

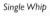

Step Back to Repulse Monkey

In this lengthy sequence, you step backward, turning first to the right, then to left, and then to the right once more. It is a good exercise for improving coordination, balance, and awareness, and it also helps to loosen the ankle joints. Make sure that you keep your alignment as you step back—remember to tuck in the chin and the tail bone. When stepping backward, always place the toes down first.

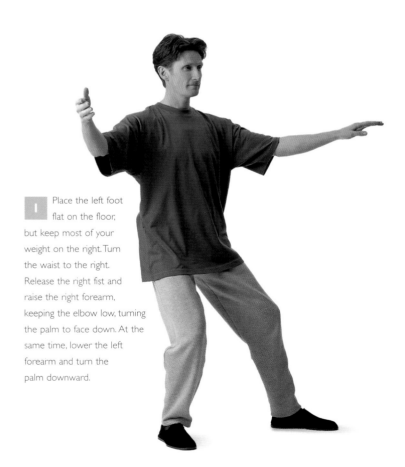

1 Place the left foot flat on the floor, but keep most of your weight on the right. Turn the waist to the right. Release the right fist and raise the right forearm, keeping the elbow low, turning the palm to face down. At the same time, lower the left forearm and turn the palm downward.

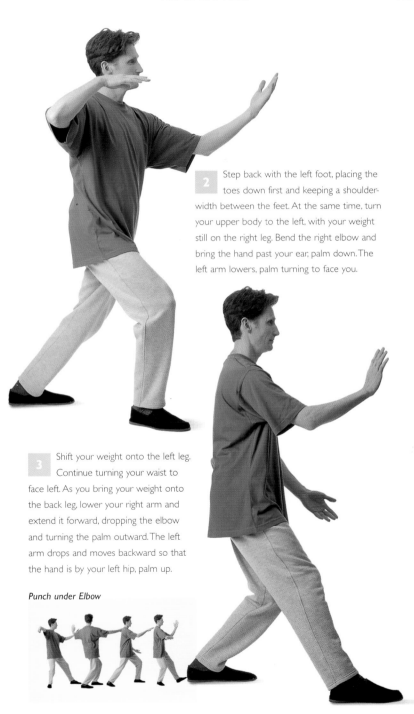

2 Step back with the left foot, placing the toes down first and keeping a shoulder-width between the feet. At the same time, turn your upper body to the left, with your weight still on the right leg. Bend the right elbow and bring the hand past your ear, palm down. The left arm lowers, palm turning to face you.

3 Shift your weight onto the left leg. Continue turning your waist to face left. As you bring your weight onto the back leg, lower your right arm and extend it forward, dropping the elbow and turning the palm outward. The left arm drops and moves backward so that the hand is by your left hip, palm up.

Punch under Elbow

Step Back to Repulse Monkey (Left)

You now repeat the movements. This time you turn to the left and step back with the right foot As you become more familiar with stepping back, try to bring a flowing rhythmic quality to your movements.

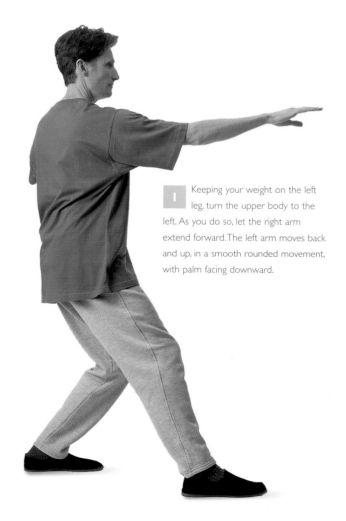

I Keeping your weight on the left leg, turn the upper body to the left. As you do so, let the right arm extend forward. The left arm moves back and up, in a smooth rounded movement, with palm facing downward.

2 Keeping the weight on the left leg, step back with the right foot, placing the toes down first and keeping it facing in the same direction as the left one. There should still be a shoulder-width distance between your feet. Bend the left arm, bringing the hand level with your ear, palm turned down. The right elbow drops and the right palm turns to face you.

3 Now bring your weight onto the right leg. Turn your upper body to the right. Slightly lower your left arm and extend it forward, dropping the elbow and turning the palm outward. The right arm drops down to your hip. Your weight should be almost entirely on the right leg.

Step Back to Repulse Monkey

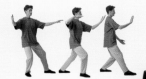

Step Back to Repulse Monkey (Right)

In the final part of the Repulse Monkey sequence, you turn to the right and step back with the left foot again. Try to synchronize all your movements so that the arms and legs move in perfect harmony.

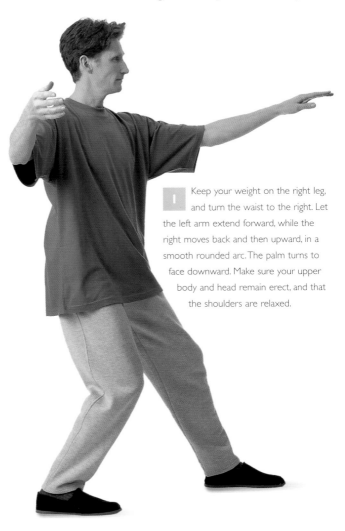

1 Keep your weight on the right leg, and turn the waist to the right. Let the left arm extend forward, while the right moves back and then upward, in a smooth rounded arc. The palm turns to face downward. Make sure your upper body and head remain erect, and that the shoulders are relaxed.

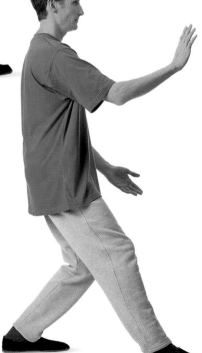

2 Keeping the weight on the right leg, step back with the left foot, placing the toes down first. There should be a shoulder-width between your feet. Keep your weight on the right leg and turn your waist to the left as you step. Bend the right elbow and bring the hand level with your ear, palm facing down. Turn the left palm to face you.

3 Move your weight onto the left leg. Continue turning your waist to the left. At the same time, lower your right arm and extend it forward, dropping the elbow and turning the palm to face away from you. The left arm drops and moves back to bring the hand to the hip, palm up. End with almost all your weight on the left leg.

Step Back *to Repulse Monkey (Left)*

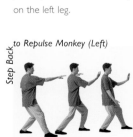

Diagonal Flying

Diagonal Flying provides a good stretch for the waist, but take care that you do not turn so far that you distort your posture. With regular practice, your waist will become more flexible and you will be able to go farther. This sequence ends with a wonderfully expansive posture, shown overleaf, that extends the whole body.

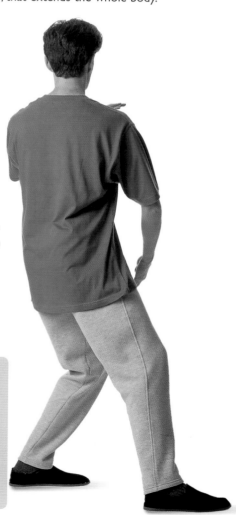

1 With most of your weight on the left leg, turn the upper body as far left as you can comfortably go. Watch that you do not twist the right knee round as you turn. At the same time, lower the right arm, turning the palm upward. Bring the left arm up in front of your chest, palm facing down. Hold the ball.

SINKING

Tai chi teachers talk about "sinking" into a posture. This means aligning the body correctly so your legs take your weight. It also means releasing any tension in the body. Always try to sink into the final pose of a sequence before moving into the next.

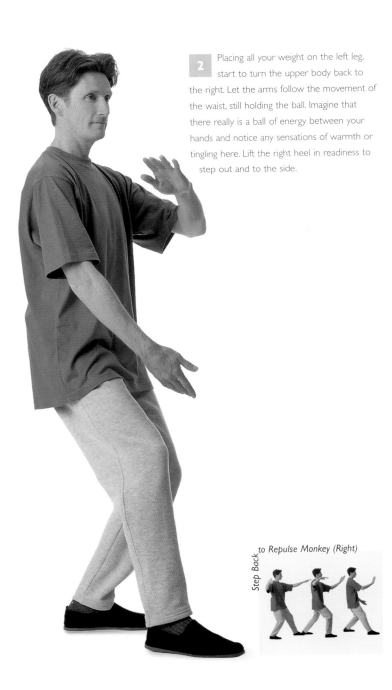

2 Placing all your weight on the left leg, start to turn the upper body back to the right. Let the arms follow the movement of the waist, still holding the ball. Imagine that there really is a ball of energy between your hands and notice any sensations of warmth or tingling here. Lift the right heel in readiness to step out and to the side.

Step Back to Repulse Monkey (Right)

Diagonal Flying

The Diagonal Flying sequence continues with a big step to the right. Watch for the tendency to lunge here—keep your weight back and step in a slow and controlled way.

1 Still holding the ball, step the right foot out to the right, placing the heel down first. Turn the upper body to the right as you step.

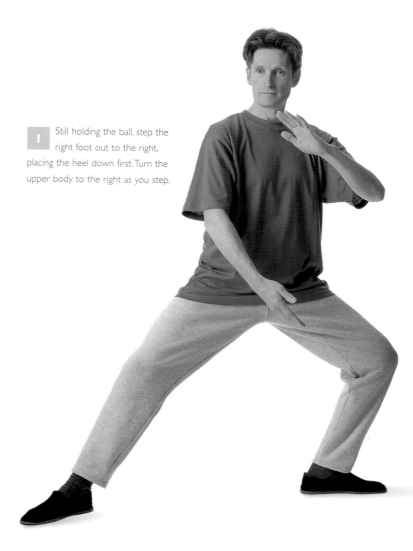

2 Keeping the spine and head erect, shift about 70 percent of your weight onto the right leg. Turn your left toes inward, to complete the bow and arrow stance. Continue turning to the right and let the right arm come up and extend outward, palm facing up. The left arm drops, palm facing backward. Your gaze is directed at the right hand.

Diagonal Flying

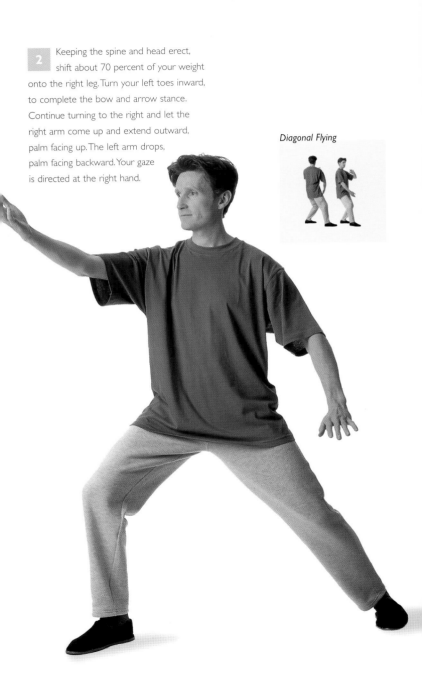

Wave Hands Like Clouds (i)

This is the start of an extended sequence that gently works the whole body. It is a favorite of many tai chi practitioners. The emphasis is on the hands, which make soft circular movements as if drawing pictures of clouds in the air. The arm movements are coordinated with turns of the upper body and the shifts in your body weight.

1 Keeping the weight on the right leg, lift the left heel. Turn on the ball to bring the left foot to face forward. As the same time, raise your right hand and lower the left. Bend both arms at the elbows, and hold the ball.

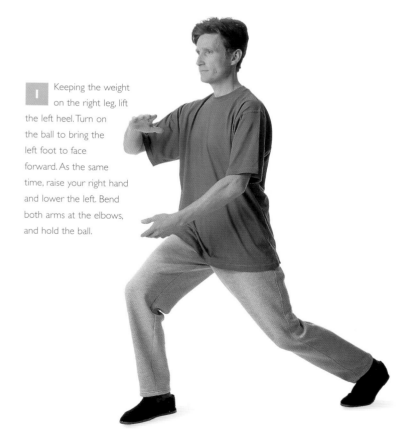

2 Move the left foot forward to bring it in line with the right foot. The distance between them should be about one and a half times the width of your shoulders. Place the heel down first. As you step, drop your right arm to hip level, palm facing your body, and raise the left arm to just below shoulder-level, palm also facing inward. The right hand passes over the left one, which remains close to the body.

3 Bring your weight onto the left leg and turn the upper body as far left as you can comfortably go. Lift the right toes and pivot on the heel to bring the foot to face forward. It should now be parallel with the left. As you turn, rotate the wrists to hold the ball again. About 70 percent of your weight should now be on the left foot. Make sure that the upper body is erect. This concludes the first part of the sequence.

Diagonal Flying

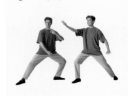

Wave Hands Like Clouds (ii)

You now continue to turn from left to right and back again, sweeping the upper hand down and the lower hand up as you turn. Enjoy the gentle rhythmic flow of the movements, and try to feel the ball of energy between the palms of your hands.

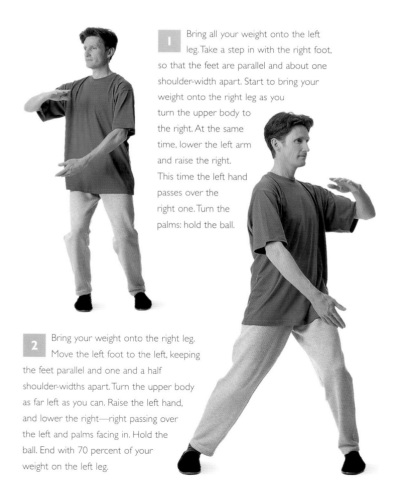

1 Bring all your weight onto the left leg. Take a step in with the right foot, so that the feet are parallel and about one shoulder-width apart. Start to bring your weight onto the right leg as you turn the upper body to the right. At the same time, lower the left arm and raise the right. This time the left hand passes over the right one. Turn the palms: hold the ball.

2 Bring your weight onto the right leg. Move the left foot to the left, keeping the feet parallel and one and a half shoulder-widths apart. Turn the upper body as far left as you can. Raise the left hand, and lower the right—right passing over the left and palms facing in. Hold the ball. End with 70 percent of your weight on the left leg.

3 Bring all your weight onto the left leg. Take an inward step with the right foot so that the feet are parallel to each other and about one shoulder-width apart. Bring your weight onto the right foot and turn the upper body to the right. At the same time, lower the left arm and raise the right, elbows bent and palms facing in. This time, the left hand passes over the right. Turn the palms to hold the ball.

4 Bring your weight onto the right leg. Step the left foot out, keeping the feet parallel. They should now be one and a half shoulder-widths apart. Turn the upper body left, as the left arm rises and the right one falls. The palms face in and the right hand passes over the left. Hold the ball. End with 70 percent of your weight on the left leg.

Wave Hands Like Clouds (i)

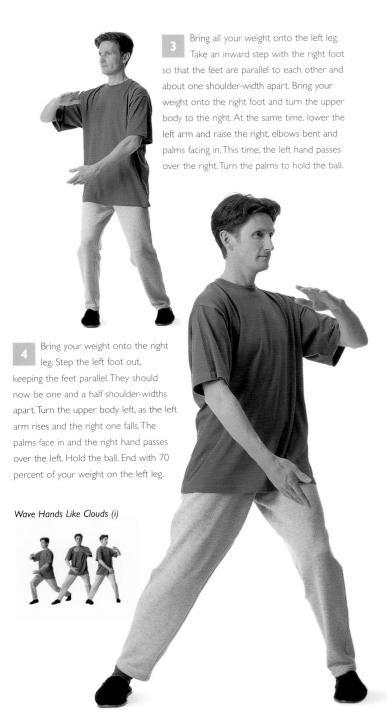

Single Whip

You now move into Single Whip once more. This is the third appearance of the sequence but this time it leads into a graceful adaptation of the final pose—Descending Single Whip. Keep your breathing soft and smooth. This will help to bring lightness to your movements.

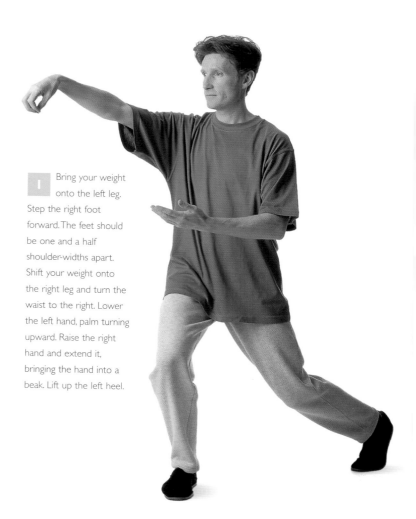

1 Bring your weight onto the left leg. Step the right foot forward. The feet should be one and a half shoulder-widths apart. Shift your weight onto the right leg and turn the waist to the right. Lower the left hand, palm turning upward. Raise the right hand and extend it, bringing the hand into a beak. Lift up the left heel.

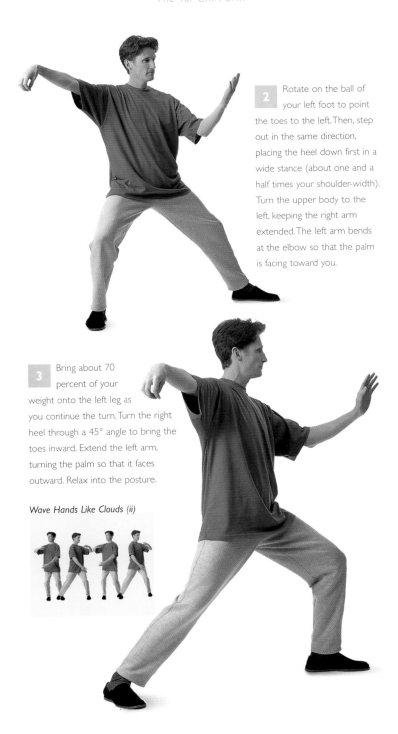

2 Rotate on the ball of your left foot to point the toes to the left. Then, step out in the same direction, placing the heel down first in a wide stance (about one and a half times your shoulder-width). Turn the upper body to the left, keeping the right arm extended. The left arm bends at the elbow so that the palm is facing toward you.

3 Bring about 70 percent of your weight onto the left leg as you continue the turn. Turn the right heel through a 45° angle to bring the toes inward. Extend the left arm, turning the palm so that it faces outward. Relax into the posture.

Wave Hands Like Clouds (ii)

Descending Single Whip

In this variation of Single Whip, you sink down in a graceful movement. This can be quite difficult unless you are very flexible. Do not try to go too far and be sure to keep your back straight. Make sure that you do not bend your knee so far that it extends over your toes.

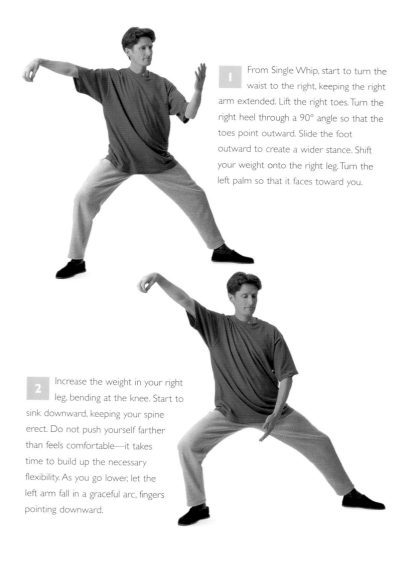

1 From Single Whip, start to turn the waist to the right, keeping the right arm extended. Lift the right toes. Turn the right heel through a 90° angle so that the toes point outward. Slide the foot outward to create a wider stance. Shift your weight onto the right leg. Turn the left palm so that it faces toward you.

2 Increase the weight in your right leg, bending at the knee. Start to sink downward, keeping your spine erect. Do not push yourself farther than feels comfortable—it takes time to build up the necessary flexibility. As you go lower, let the left arm fall in a graceful arc, fingers pointing downward.

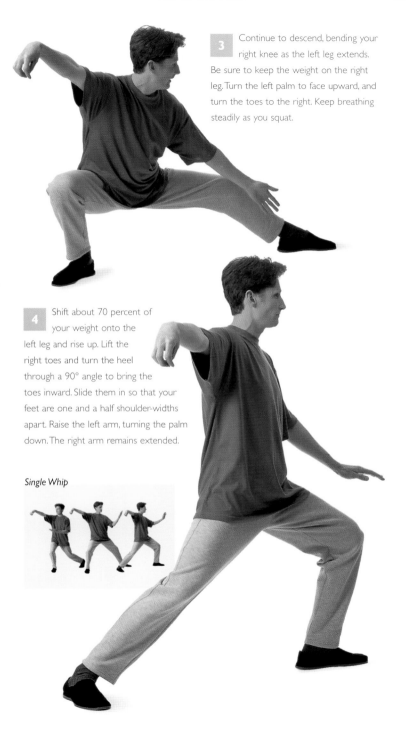

3 Continue to descend, bending your right knee as the left leg extends. Be sure to keep the weight on the right leg. Turn the left palm to face upward, and turn the toes to the right. Keep breathing steadily as you squat.

4 Shift about 70 percent of your weight onto the left leg and rise up. Lift the right toes and turn the heel through a 90° angle to bring the toes inward. Slide them in so that your feet are one and a half shoulder-widths apart. Raise the left arm, turning the palm down. The right arm remains extended.

Single Whip

Golden Rooster Stands on Left Leg

This sequence requires good balance and stability. It will help if you look straight ahead when standing on one leg—find a point on the wall to focus on. If you find this pose difficult, leave the toes resting on the ground rather than raising the leg. Focus on keeping all your weight in the left leg. Your balance will improve with practice.

1 Bring almost all your weight onto the left leg. Lower the right arm, releasing the hand from its beak and letting the fingers point downward.

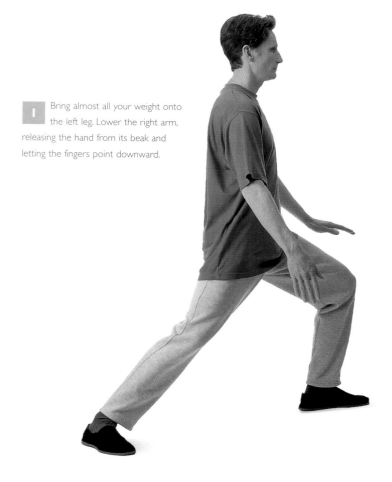

2 Shift all your weight onto the left leg, as you step the right foot forward, resting the toes near the left heel. Then, bring up the right leg, bending the knee and bringing it level with your waist or as close to it as you can comfortably go—ideally your thigh will be level with the floor. Your toes should drop downward. At the same time, raise the right arm, bending the elbow and pointing the fingers upward. The fingers of the left hand point down.

Descending Single Whip

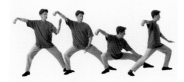

Golden Rooster Stands on Right Leg

Here you repeat the balance posture in reverse, so that you stand on the right leg and lift up the left one. Watch that you do not tense up. Keep the shoulders and hips relaxed, and the back and head erect.

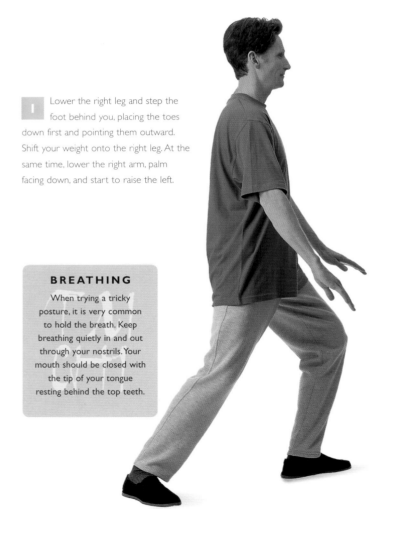

1 Lower the right leg and step the foot behind you, placing the toes down first and pointing them outward. Shift your weight onto the right leg. At the same time, lower the right arm, palm facing down, and start to raise the left.

BREATHING

When trying a tricky posture, it is very common to hold the breath. Keep breathing quietly in and out through your nostrils. Your mouth should be closed with the tip of your tongue resting behind the top teeth.

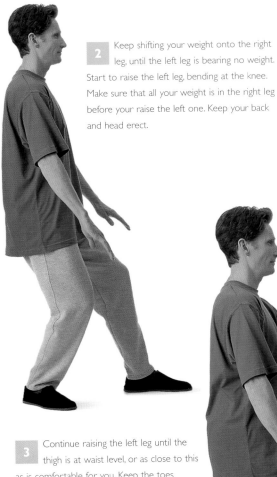

2 Keep shifting your weight onto the right leg, until the left leg is bearing no weight. Start to raise the left leg, bending at the knee. Make sure that all your weight is in the right leg before your raise the left one. Keep your back and head erect.

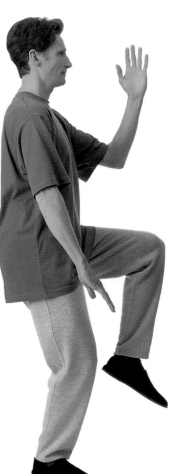

3 Continue raising the left leg until the thigh is at waist level, or as close to this as is comfortable for you. Keep the toes pointing downward. The right arm stays dropped, fingers pointing to the ground. Lift the left forearm, keeping the elbow dropped down. The fingers should point upward.

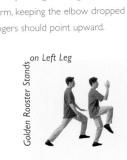

Golden Rooster Stands on Left Leg

Right Toe Kick

This sequence involves another balance pose, this time a kick which helps to stretch the front of the leg. Do not kick the leg too high, and remember to keep the movement slow and controlled.

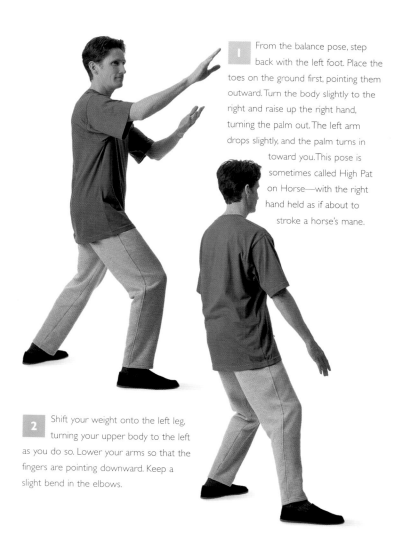

1 From the balance pose, step back with the left foot. Place the toes on the ground first, pointing them outward. Turn the body slightly to the right and raise up the right hand, turning the palm out. The left arm drops slightly, and the palm turns in toward you. This pose is sometimes called High Pat on Horse—with the right hand held as if about to stroke a horse's mane.

2 Shift your weight onto the left leg, turning your upper body to the left as you do so. Lower your arms so that the fingers are pointing downward. Keep a slight bend in the elbows.

3 Keep turning to the left, and bring the rest of your weight onto the left leg. Draw in the right foot, placing it next to the left one. Keep the heel raised. At the same time, raise the arms up the center of the body, crossing the right wrist over the left one. Your palms should be facing toward you.

4 Turn the waist to the right. Open out the arms, turning the palms outward. Raise the left forearm and lower the right one. Then move all your weight onto the left leg. Raise the right foot into a kick, pointing the toes but keeping the foot relaxed. Remember to keep the supporting leg slightly bent.

Golden Rooster Stands on Right Leg

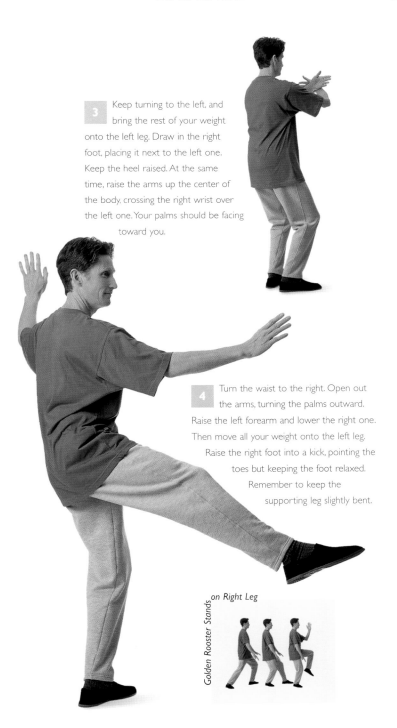

Left Toe Kick

Now you repeat the kick with the left leg. Remain aware of the
tan tien (energy center), in your lower abdomen, and let the movement
unfold from here. This will help you move in a conscious way.

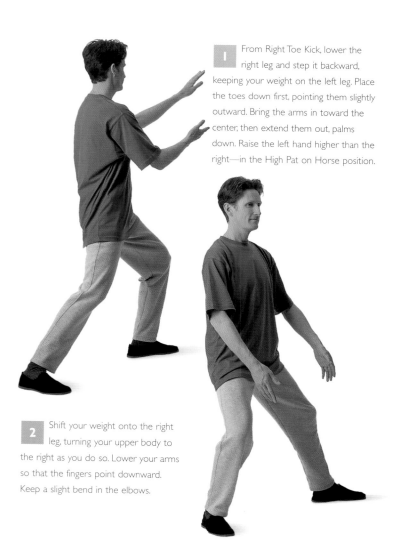

1 From Right Toe Kick, lower the
right leg and step it backward,
keeping your weight on the left leg. Place
the toes down first, pointing them slightly
outward. Bring the arms in toward the
center, then extend them out, palms
down. Raise the left hand higher than the
right—in the High Pat on Horse position.

2 Shift your weight onto the right
leg, turning your upper body to
the right as you do so. Lower your arms
so that the fingers point downward.
Keep a slight bend in the elbows.

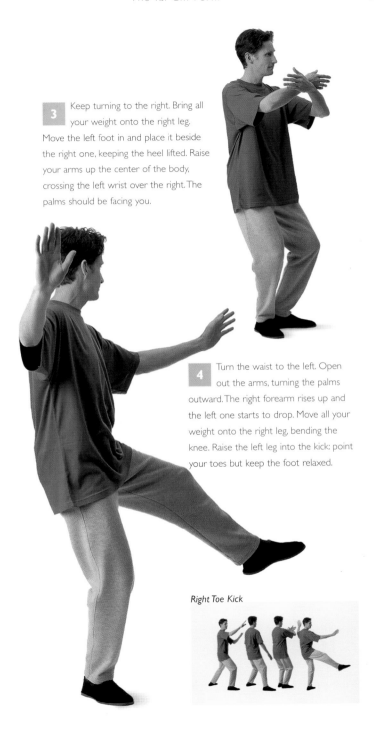

3 Keep turning to the right. Bring all your weight onto the right leg. Move the left foot in and place it beside the right one, keeping the heel lifted. Raise your arms up the center of the body, crossing the left wrist over the right. The palms should be facing you.

4 Turn the waist to the left. Open out the arms, turning the palms outward. The right forearm rises up and the left one starts to drop. Move all your weight onto the right leg, bending the knee. Raise the left leg into the kick: point your toes but keep the foot relaxed.

Right Toe Kick

Turn and Kick with Left Heel

In this movement, you turn the body through a semi-circle from left to right, pivoting all the way on the right heel. Your turn will become smoother with practice. If you find it difficult to balance, bring the left toes to rest on the ground behind the right heel. Use them to stabilize yourself during the turn.

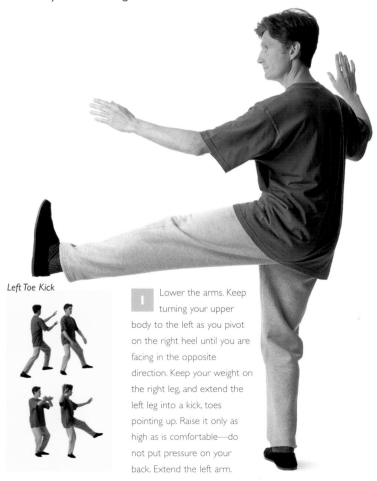

Left Toe Kick

1 Lower the arms. Keep turning your upper body to the left as you pivot on the right heel until you are facing in the opposite direction. Keep your weight on the right leg, and extend the left leg into a kick, toes pointing up. Raise it only as high as is comfortable—do not put pressure on your back. Extend the left arm.

Brush Left Knee and Push

This is the third time that the Brush Left Knee and Push sequence appears in the form. This time, you start from a kick, so the left leg is raised. Take care that you do not fall or lean into the first movement. Lower the left leg with control and keep your weight on the right leg.

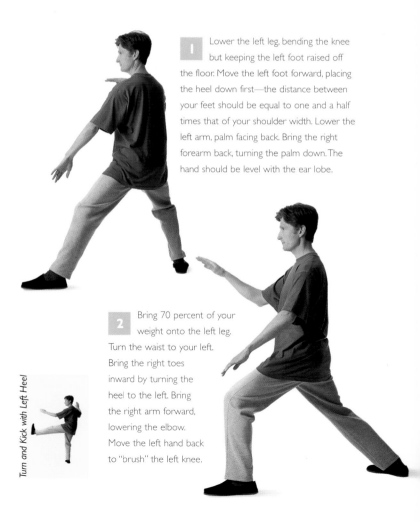

1 Lower the left leg, bending the knee but keeping the left foot raised off the floor. Move the left foot forward, placing the heel down first—the distance between your feet should be equal to one and a half times that of your shoulder width. Lower the left arm, palm facing back. Bring the right forearm back, turning the palm down. The hand should be level with the ear lobe.

2 Bring 70 percent of your weight onto the left leg. Turn the waist to your left. Bring the right toes inward by turning the heel to the left. Bring the right arm forward, lowering the elbow. Move the left hand back to "brush" the left knee.

Turn and Kick with Left Heel

Brush Right
Knee and Push

Now you repeat the Brush Knee sequence with the other side. In tai
chi, you often mirror a movement to help keep the body balanced. The
circling movement of the arms helps to open the chest.

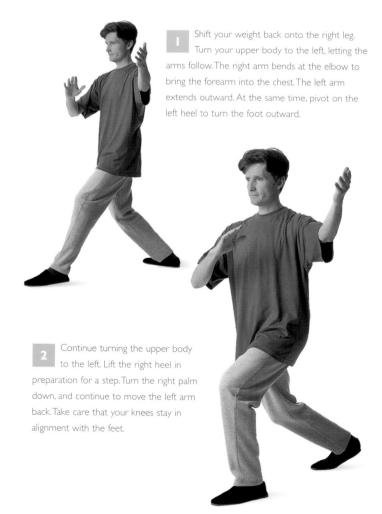

1 Shift your weight back onto the right leg.
Turn your upper body to the left, letting the
arms follow. The right arm bends at the elbow to
bring the forearm into the chest. The left arm
extends outward. At the same time, pivot on the
left heel to turn the foot outward.

2 Continue turning the upper body
to the left. Lift the right heel in
preparation for a step. Turn the right palm
down, and continue to move the left arm
back. Take care that your knees stay in
alignment with the feet.

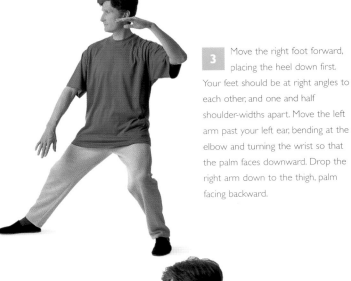

3 Move the right foot forward, placing the heel down first. Your feet should be at right angles to each other, and one and half shoulder-widths apart. Move the left arm past your left ear, bending at the elbow and turning the wrist so that the palm faces downward. Drop the right arm down to the thigh, palm facing backward.

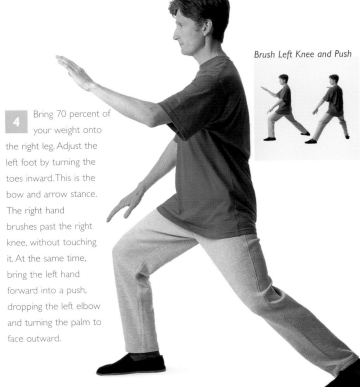

Brush Left Knee and Push

4 Bring 70 percent of your weight onto the right leg. Adjust the left foot by turning the toes inward. This is the bow and arrow stance. The right hand brushes past the right knee, without touching it. At the same time, bring the left hand forward into a push, dropping the left elbow and turning the palm to face outward.

Brush Left Knee and Punch Downward

Here you brush the left knee once again, but this time you throw a low punch with the right hand. Do not lean forward in the final posture; keep your back straight and go only as far as is comfortable. This exercise improves flexibility in the lower back.

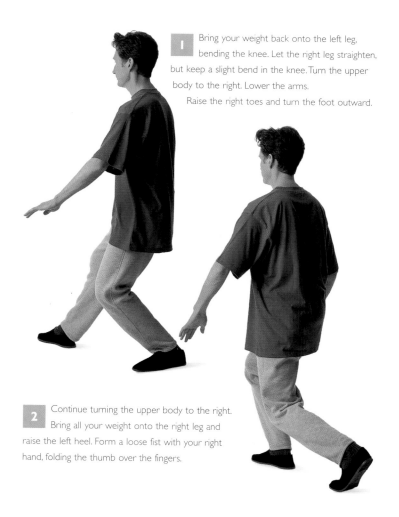

I Bring your weight back onto the left leg, bending the knee. Let the right leg straighten, but keep a slight bend in the knee. Turn the upper body to the right. Lower the arms.

Raise the right toes and turn the foot outward.

2 Continue turning the upper body to the right. Bring all your weight onto the right leg and raise the left heel. Form a loose fist with your right hand, folding the thumb over the fingers.

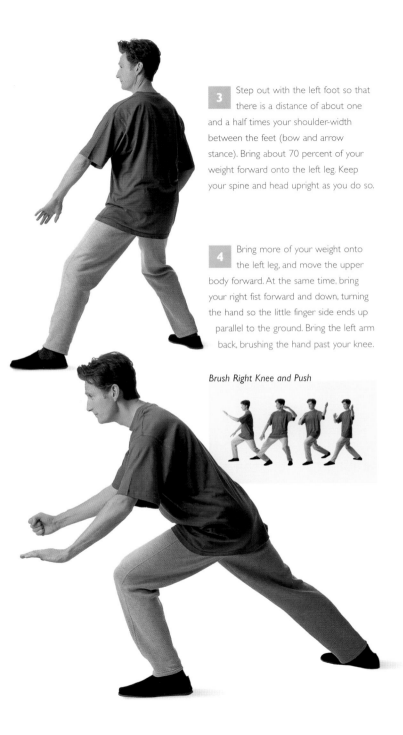

3 Step out with the left foot so that there is a distance of about one and a half times your shoulder-width between the feet (bow and arrow stance). Bring about 70 percent of your weight forward onto the left leg. Keep your spine and head upright as you do so.

4 Bring more of your weight onto the left leg, and move the upper body forward. At the same time, bring your right fist forward and down, turning the hand so the little finger side ends up parallel to the ground. Bring the left arm back, brushing the hand past your knee.

Brush Right Knee and Push

Ward Off Right

This is the second time that Ward Off Right has appeared in the form and it heralds the start of an extended sequence of familiar movements. This time there is an extra move at the beginning, which is needed to bring you up from the low stance of the punch.

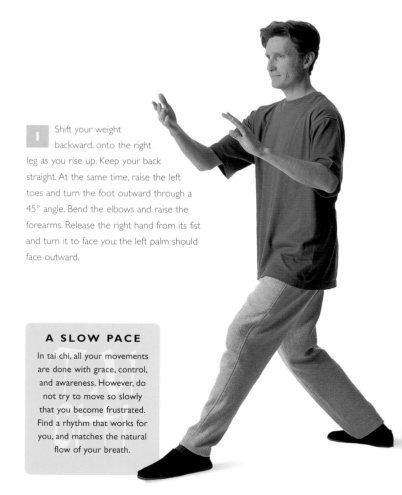

1 Shift your weight backward, onto the right leg as you rise up. Keep your back straight. At the same time, raise the left toes and turn the foot outward through a 45° angle. Bend the elbows and raise the forearms. Release the right hand from its fist and turn it to face you; the left palm should face outward.

A SLOW PACE

In tai chi, all your movements are done with grace, control, and awareness. However, do not try to move so slowly that you become frustrated. Find a rhythm that works for you, and matches the natural flow of your breath.

2 Bring your weight onto the left leg and turn the upper body to the left. Let the right heel rise off the ground. The arms continue to rise up.

3 Move the right foot forward so that the feet are one and a half shoulder-widths apart. Place the heel down first. As you step, turn the upper body to the right. Your left arm folds inward, so that fingers point toward the right wrist. Shift your weight as you turn, to end with 70 percent of it on the right leg. This is the bow and arrow stance again.

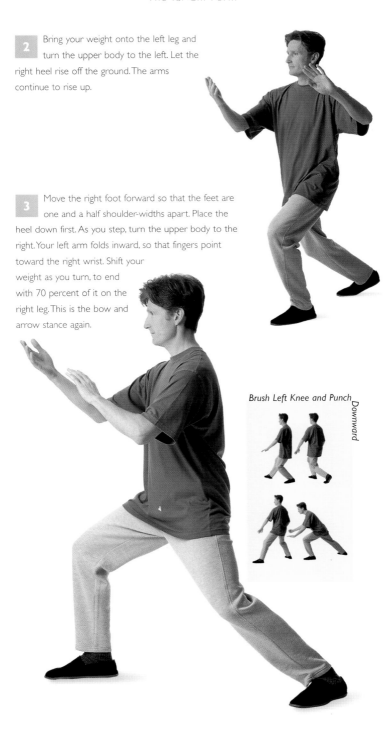

Brush Left Knee and Punch Downward

Rollback

Here, the repetition of Rollback provides an opportunity to bring energy back into the body. Keep breathing softly through the nostrils as you move—do not hold your breath at any point.

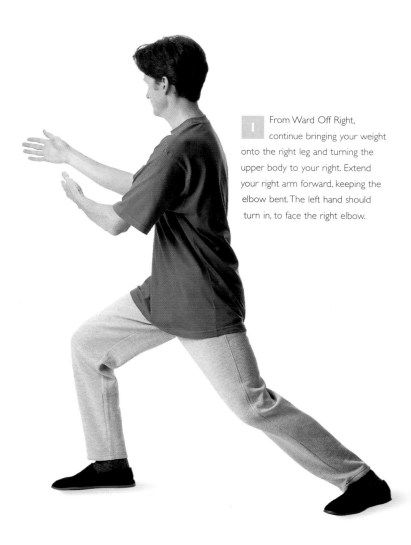

1 From Ward Off Right, continue bringing your weight onto the right leg and turning the upper body to your right. Extend your right arm forward, keeping the elbow bent. The left hand should turn in, to face the right elbow.

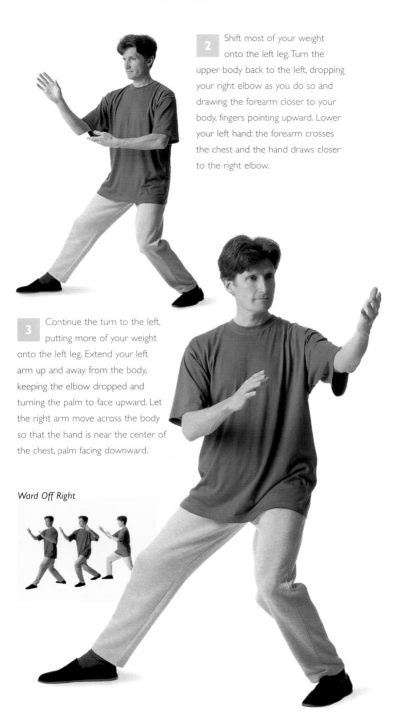

2 Shift most of your weight onto the left leg. Turn the upper body back to the left, dropping your right elbow as you do so and drawing the forearm closer to your body, fingers pointing upward. Lower your left hand: the forearm crosses the chest and the hand draws closer to the right elbow.

3 Continue the turn to the left, putting more of your weight onto the left leg. Extend your left arm up and away from the body, keeping the elbow dropped and turning the palm to face upward. Let the right arm move across the body so that the hand is near the center of the chest, palm facing downward.

Ward Off Right

Press and Push

You glide smoothly from Rollback into Press and Push. Enjoy the familiarity of these movements, practiced here for the third time in the form, but remember to keep your mental focus at all times.

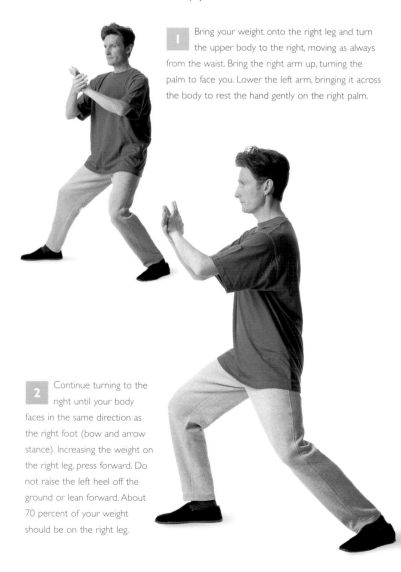

1 Bring your weight onto the right leg and turn the upper body to the right, moving as always from the waist. Bring the right arm up, turning the palm to face you. Lower the left arm, bringing it across the body to rest the hand gently on the right palm.

2 Continue turning to the right until your body faces in the same direction as the right foot (bow and arrow stance). Increasing the weight on the right leg, press forward. Do not raise the left heel off the ground or lean forward. About 70 percent of your weight should be on the right leg.

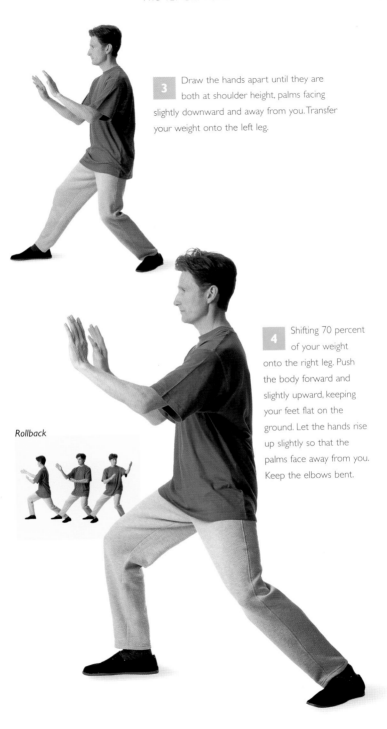

3 Draw the hands apart until they are both at shoulder height, palms facing slightly downward and away from you. Transfer your weight onto the left leg.

4 Shifting 70 percent of your weight onto the right leg. Push the body forward and slightly upward, keeping your feet flat on the ground. Let the hands rise up slightly so that the palms face away from you. Keep the elbows bent.

Rollback

Single Whip

Here as before, you move into Single Whip from the Push position. Keep your back and head erect. It will help if you imagine that you are held upright by a thread attached to the crown of your head.

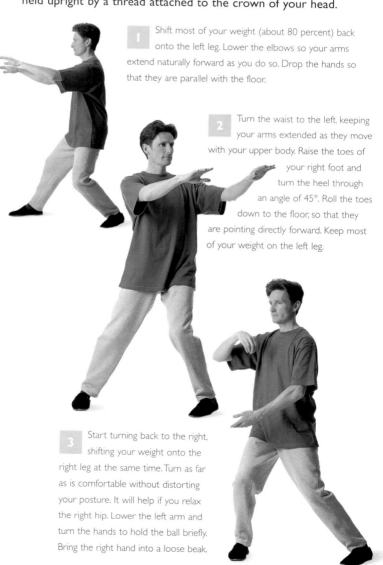

1 Shift most of your weight (about 80 percent) back onto the left leg. Lower the elbows so your arms extend naturally forward as you do so. Drop the hands so that they are parallel with the floor.

2 Turn the waist to the left, keeping your arms extended as they move with your upper body. Raise the toes of your right foot and turn the heel through an angle of 45°. Roll the toes down to the floor, so that they are pointing directly forward. Keep most of your weight on the left leg.

3 Start turning back to the right, shifting your weight onto the right leg at the same time. Turn as far as is comfortable without distorting your posture. It will help if you relax the right hip. Lower the left arm and turn the hands to hold the ball briefly. Bring the right hand into a loose beak.

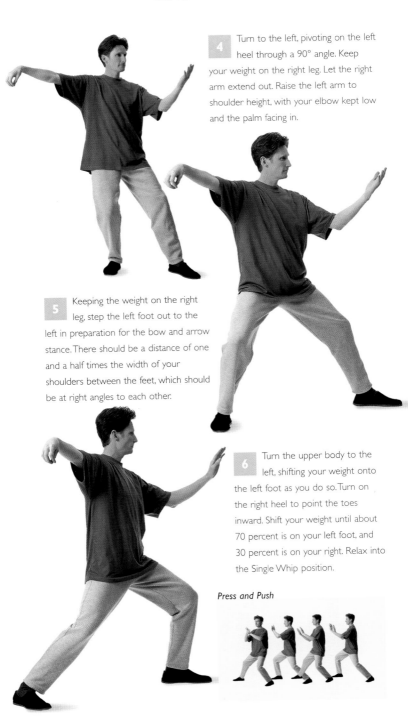

4 Turn to the left, pivoting on the left heel through a 90° angle. Keep your weight on the right leg. Let the right arm extend out. Raise the left arm to shoulder height, with your elbow kept low and the palm facing in.

5 Keeping the weight on the right leg, step the left foot out to the left in preparation for the bow and arrow stance. There should be a distance of one and a half times the width of your shoulders between the feet, which should be at right angles to each other.

6 Turn the upper body to the left, shifting your weight onto the left foot as you do so. Turn on the right heel to point the toes inward. Shift your weight until about 70 percent is on your left foot, and 30 percent is on your right. Relax into the Single Whip position.

Press and Push

Fair Lady Weaves the Shuttle (i)

Fair Lady Weaves the Shuttle is a delightful, but lengthy sequence. It gets its name from the actions of the hands, which open and close as if using a loom. The same movements are performed four times, but the body faces in a different direction each time. The sequence is sometimes known as Four Corners for this reason.

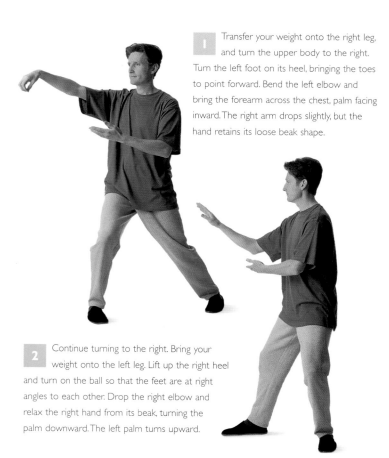

1 Transfer your weight onto the right leg, and turn the upper body to the right. Turn the left foot on its heel, bringing the toes to point forward. Bend the left elbow and bring the forearm across the chest, palm facing inward. The right arm drops slightly, but the hand retains its loose beak shape.

2 Continue turning to the right. Bring your weight onto the left leg. Lift up the right heel and turn on the ball so that the feet are at right angles to each other. Drop the right elbow and relax the right hand from its beak, turning the palm downward. The left palm turns upward.

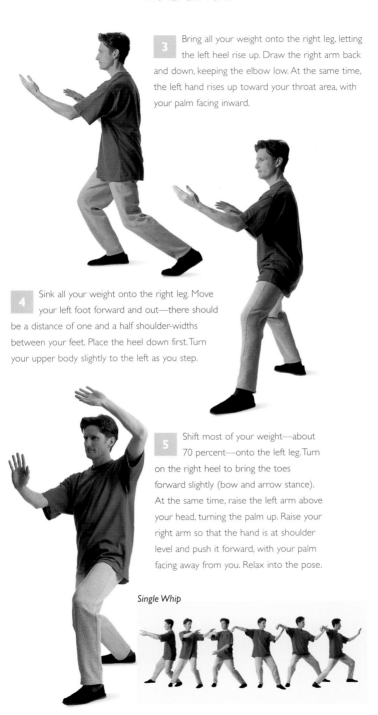

3 Bring all your weight onto the right leg, letting the left heel rise up. Draw the right arm back and down, keeping the elbow low. At the same time, the left hand rises up toward your throat area, with your palm facing inward.

4 Sink all your weight onto the right leg. Move your left foot forward and out—there should be a distance of one and a half shoulder-widths between your feet. Place the heel down first. Turn your upper body slightly to the left as you step.

5 Shift most of your weight—about 70 percent—onto the left leg. Turn on the right heel to bring the toes forward slightly (bow and arrow stance). At the same time, raise the left arm above your head, turning the palm up. Raise your right arm so that the hand is at shoulder level and push it forward, with your palm facing away from you. Relax into the pose.

Single Whip

Fair Lady Weaves the Shuttle (ii)

Move smoothly into the second set of movements. This involves making a large clockwise turn through three-quarters of a circle, so that you turn to the right but end up facing left.

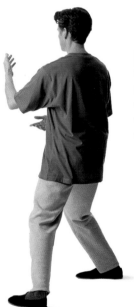

1 Bring all your weight onto the right leg. Lower the arms. Turn the left palm in to face you, and the right palm upward, near to the left elbow. At the same time, raise the left toes and turn the heel through a 90° angle to your right.

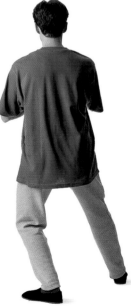

2 Now bring almost all of your weight onto the left leg. Raise the right heel and turn the ball of the foot through a 90° angle. At the same time, turn the body to the right. Start to lower the left forearm and raise the right forearm as you turn. The right palm turns to face you. The left palm faces down.

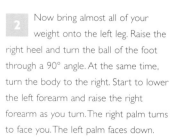

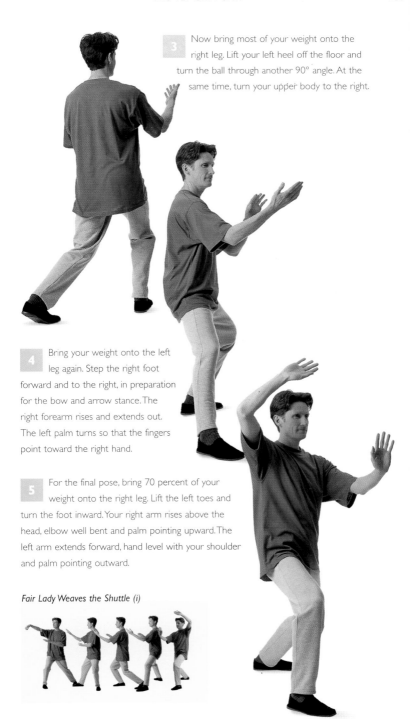

3 Now bring most of your weight onto the right leg. Lift your left heel off the floor and turn the ball through another 90° angle. At the same time, turn your upper body to the right.

4 Bring your weight onto the left leg again. Step the right foot forward and to the right, in preparation for the bow and arrow stance. The right forearm rises and extends out. The left palm turns so that the fingers point toward the right hand.

5 For the final pose, bring 70 percent of your weight onto the right leg. Lift the left toes and turn the foot inward. Your right arm rises above the head, elbow well bent and palm pointing upward. The left arm extends forward, hand level with your shoulder and palm pointing outward.

Fair Lady Weaves the Shuttle (i)

Fair Lady Weaves the Shuttle (iii)

You now turn the body left, to face the third of the four corners. Keep the wrists, elbows, and shoulder joints relaxed, to ensure that your arm movements are soft and flowing.

1 Bring your weight onto the left leg. Turn the upper body to the left. At the same time, turn the left palm in to face you, and lower the right forearm, turning the palm away from you. The left palm should point to the right elbow. Raise the right heel and turn the foot inward through a 45° angle. Place it flat on the floor again.

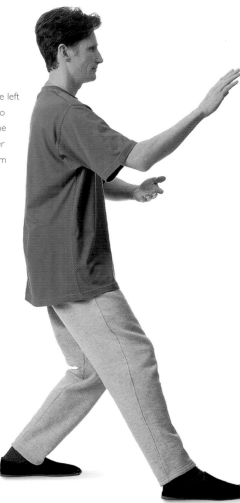

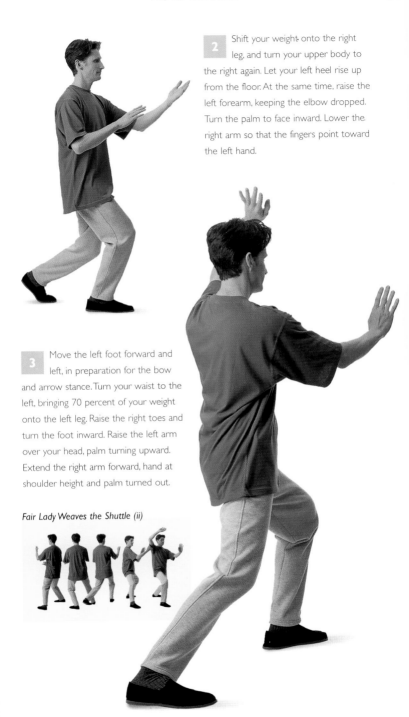

2 Shift your weight onto the right leg, and turn your upper body to the right again. Let your left heel rise up from the floor. At the same time, raise the left forearm, keeping the elbow dropped. Turn the palm to face inward. Lower the right arm so that the fingers point toward the left hand.

3 Move the left foot forward and left, in preparation for the bow and arrow stance. Turn your waist to the left, bringing 70 percent of your weight onto the left leg. Raise the right toes and turn the foot inward. Raise the left arm over your head, palm turning upward. Extend the right arm forward, hand at shoulder height and palm turned out.

Fair Lady Weaves the Shuttle (ii)

Fair Lady Weaves the Shuttle (iv)

The final part of the sequence involves another turn of 270°, again in a clockwise direction. If you are finding it hard to work out which arm to raise, bear in mind that it is always the side with the leading leg.

1 Bring your weight onto the right leg, and turn your upper body to the right. Lift the left heel and turn the foot through a 90° angle to the right. Drop the left forearm, palm turning in. Lower the right arm, dropping the elbow and turning the palm to face you.

2 Now shift your weight onto the left leg, and continue to turn your body to the right. Lift the right heel and turn the foot to the right through a 90° angle. It should now point forward. Raise the right forearm, keeping the elbow low. Let the left forearm drop, turning the palm to face down. Your left fingers should point to the right hand.

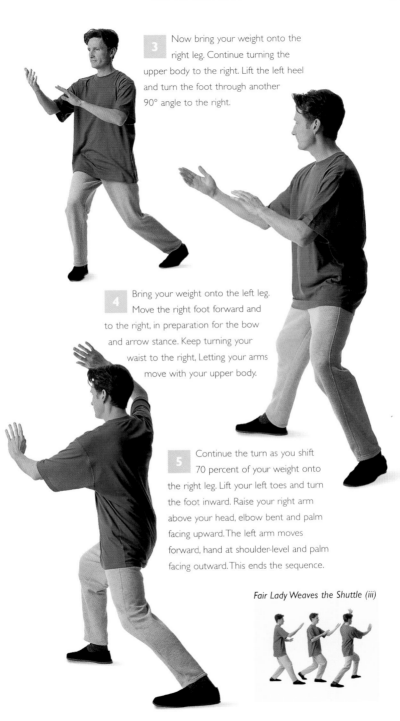

3 Now bring your weight onto the right leg. Continue turning the upper body to the right. Lift the left heel and turn the foot through another 90° angle to the right.

4 Bring your weight onto the left leg. Move the right foot forward and to the right, in preparation for the bow and arrow stance. Keep turning your waist to the right, Letting your arms move with your upper body.

5 Continue the turn as you shift 70 percent of your weight onto the right leg. Lift your left toes and turn the foot inward. Raise your right arm above your head, elbow bent and palm facing upward. The left arm moves forward, hand at shoulder-level and palm facing outward. This ends the sequence.

Fair Lady Weaves the Shuttle (iii)

Ward Off Left

From Fair Lady Weaves the Shuttle, you now move into the familiar sequence of Ward Off Left. This is a strong pose, which helps to create stability and energy for the movements that follow.

1 Move your weight onto the left leg. Raise the right toes and turn the heel so that the foot points in the same direction as the left. Turn your upper body to the left. At the same time, lower both arms and bring them into position to hold the ball—the right hand is raised with the palm facing downward while the left hand is level with the lower abdomen, palm facing upward. Bring your weight back onto the right leg.

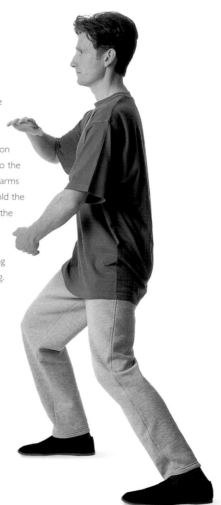

KEEP YOUR FOCUS

When performing a familiar sequence, it is easy to let your movements become automatic. Check your posture is erect and relaxed, and keep your mind focused on what you are doing.

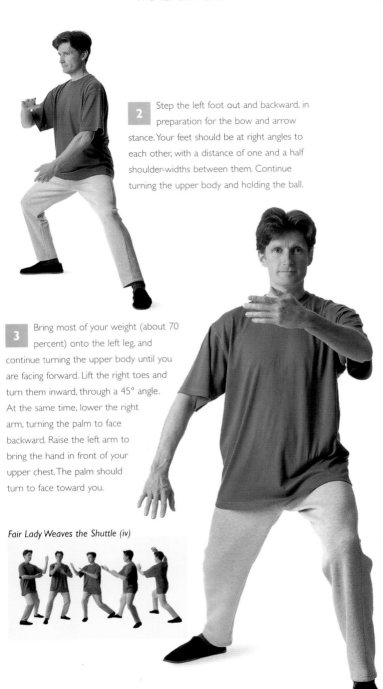

2 Step the left foot out and backward, in preparation for the bow and arrow stance. Your feet should be at right angles to each other, with a distance of one and a half shoulder-widths between them. Continue turning the upper body and holding the ball.

3 Bring most of your weight (about 70 percent) onto the left leg, and continue turning the upper body until you are facing forward. Lift the right toes and turn them inward, through a 45° angle. At the same time, lower the right arm, turning the palm to face backward. Raise the left arm to bring the hand in front of your upper chest. The palm should turn to face toward you.

Fair Lady Weaves the Shuttle (iv)

Ward Off Right

You now repeat the sequence on the right side. Ward Off Right leads
into the movements of Rollback, Press, Push, and Single Whip. This is
the fourth time that this extended sequence appears in the form.

1 Sink almost all your weight onto the
left leg and lift the right heel. Turn
your waist slightly to the left. At the
same time, move the right palm to
face upward and the left to face
downward. Hold the ball.

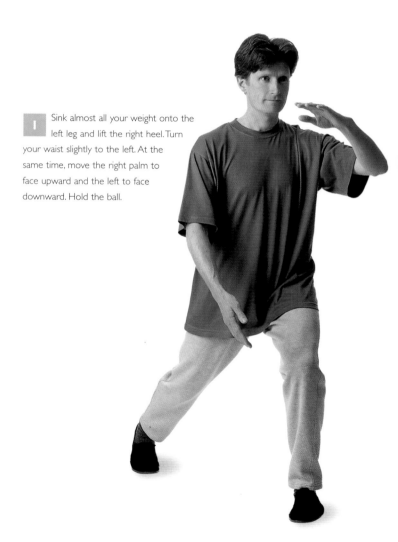

2 Turning slightly to the right, step the right foot out so that the toes point to the right. You should be in a wide stance, with a distance equal to one and a half times the width of your shoulders. Your feet should be at right angles to each other. Place the heel down first, and bend the right knee. Lower the left arm and bring the forearm across your chest, palm facing downward. The right arm rises and the forearm extends out, palm facing inward.

3 Bring about 70 percent of your weight onto the right leg. Turn at the waist until your upper body faces right. Adjust the left foot by turning on the heel through an angle of about 45°. This is the bow and arrow stance again. Move the right arm up and away from the body. Your left arm should be slightly lower, fingers pointing to the right palm.

Ward Off Left

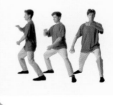

Rollback

In Rollback, the feet stay in the same position as you turn the upper body back to the right in a fluid movement. Keep the hips soft so that the waist can turn without restriction.

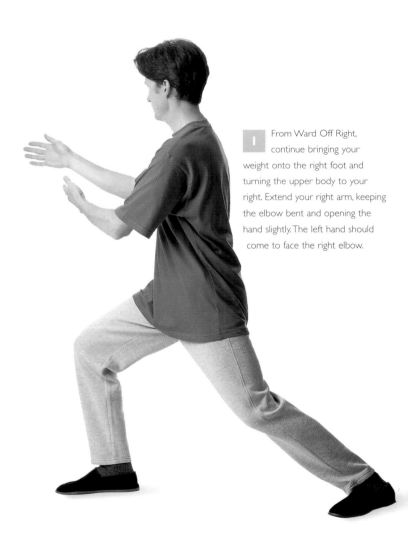

1 From Ward Off Right, continue bringing your weight onto the right foot and turning the upper body to your right. Extend your right arm, keeping the elbow bent and opening the hand slightly. The left hand should come to face the right elbow.

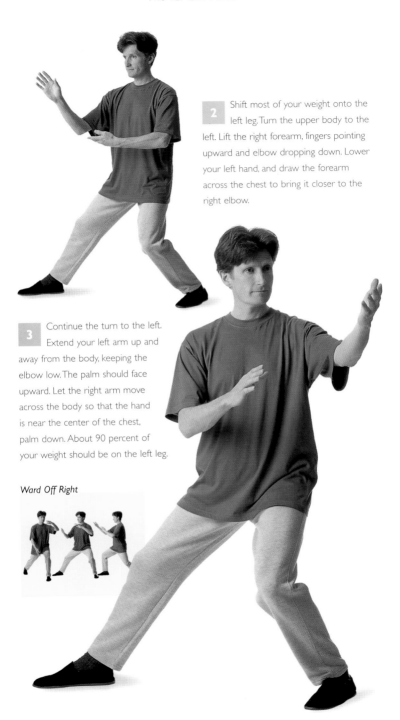

2 Shift most of your weight onto the left leg. Turn the upper body to the left. Lift the right forearm, fingers pointing upward and elbow dropping down. Lower your left hand, and draw the forearm across the chest to bring it closer to the right elbow.

3 Continue the turn to the left. Extend your left arm up and away from the body, keeping the elbow low. The palm should face upward. Let the right arm move across the body so that the hand is near the center of the chest, palm down. About 90 percent of your weight should be on the left leg.

Ward Off Right

Press and Push

As in the previous sequence, all the movement here is in the upper body—the feet remain still. Keep your upper body light as you root yourself into the ground, drawing strength and stability from it.

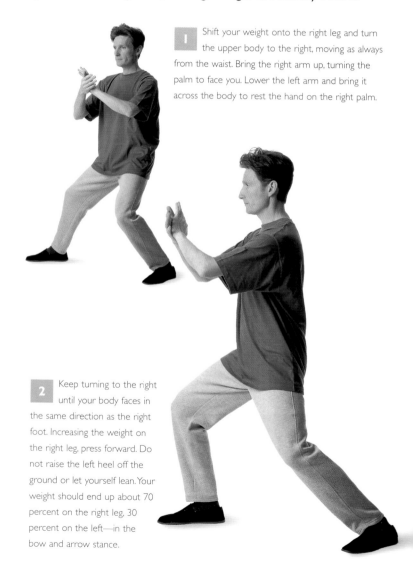

1 Shift your weight onto the right leg and turn the upper body to the right, moving as always from the waist. Bring the right arm up, turning the palm to face you. Lower the left arm and bring it across the body to rest the hand on the right palm.

2 Keep turning to the right until your body faces in the same direction as the right foot. Increasing the weight on the right leg, press forward. Do not raise the left heel off the ground or let yourself lean. Your weight should end up about 70 percent on the right leg, 30 percent on the left—in the bow and arrow stance.

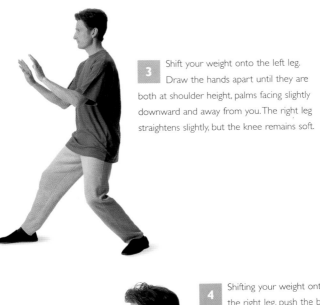

3 Shift your weight onto the left leg. Draw the hands apart until they are both at shoulder height, palms facing slightly downward and away from you. The right leg straightens slightly, but the knee remains soft.

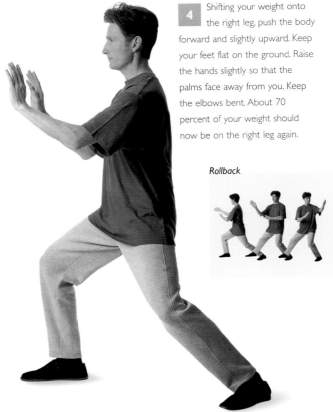

4 Shifting your weight onto the right leg, push the body forward and slightly upward. Keep your feet flat on the ground. Raise the hands slightly so that the palms face away from you. Keep the elbows bent. About 70 percent of your weight should now be on the right leg again.

Rollback

Single Whip

The body goes through many subtle adjustments in this sequence, which requires focus, balance, and control. Energy stored in the body during the previous moves is released in the final pose.

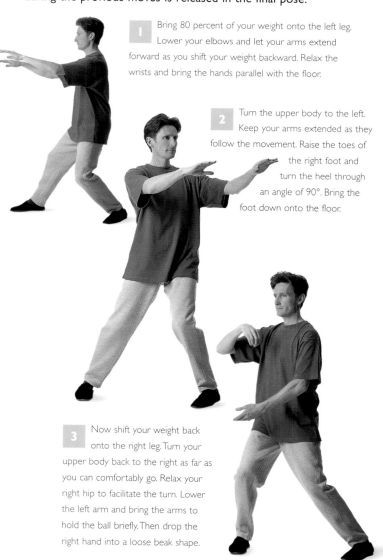

1 Bring 80 percent of your weight onto the left leg. Lower your elbows and let your arms extend forward as you shift your weight backward. Relax the wrists and bring the hands parallel with the floor.

2 Turn the upper body to the left. Keep your arms extended as they follow the movement. Raise the toes of the right foot and turn the heel through an angle of 90°. Bring the foot down onto the floor.

3 Now shift your weight back onto the right leg. Turn your upper body back to the right as far as you can comfortably go. Relax your right hip to facilitate the turn. Lower the left arm and bring the arms to hold the ball briefly. Then drop the right hand into a loose beak shape.

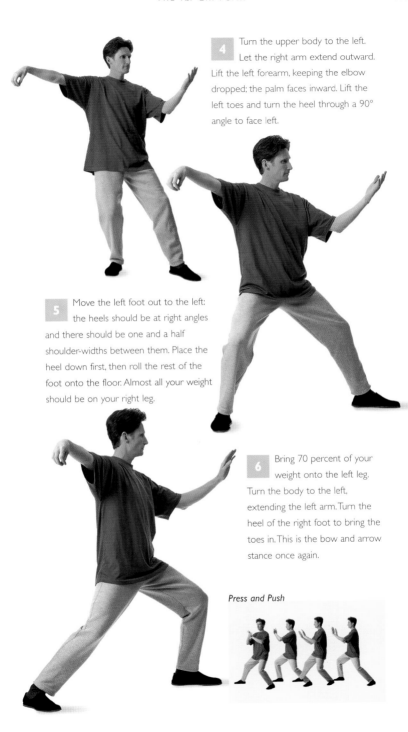

4 Turn the upper body to the left. Let the right arm extend outward. Lift the left forearm, keeping the elbow dropped; the palm faces inward. Lift the left toes and turn the heel through a 90° angle to face left.

5 Move the left foot out to the left: the heels should be at right angles and there should be one and a half shoulder-widths between them. Place the heel down first, then roll the rest of the foot onto the floor. Almost all your weight should be on your right leg.

6 Bring 70 percent of your weight onto the left leg. Turn the body to the left, extending the left arm. Turn the heel of the right foot to bring the toes in. This is the bow and arrow stance once again.

Press and Push

Descending Single Whip

This variation of Single Whip is performed here for the second time. You need good balance as well as flexibility for the squat. Do not sink lower than you can comfortably go, and keep your back straight.

1 From Single Whip, turn the upper body to the right, keeping the right arm extended with the hand still in its beak shape. Lift the right toes and turn the foot through a 90° angle to the right. Slide the foot out to create a wider stance. Shift your weight onto the right leg. Turn the left palm to face you.

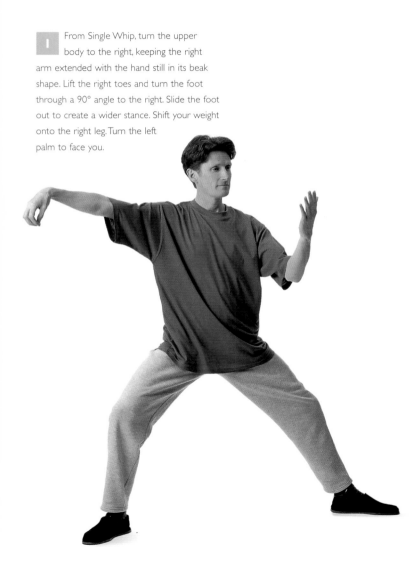

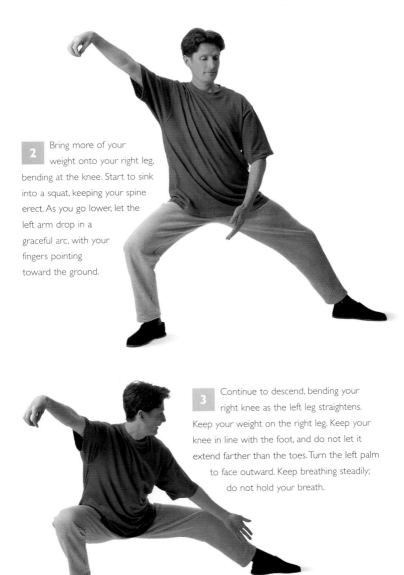

2 Bring more of your weight onto your right leg, bending at the knee. Start to sink into a squat, keeping your spine erect. As you go lower, let the left arm drop in a graceful arc, with your fingers pointing toward the ground.

3 Continue to descend, bending your right knee as the left leg straightens. Keep your weight on the right leg. Keep your knee in line with the foot, and do not let it extend farther than the toes. Turn the left palm to face outward. Keep breathing steadily; do not hold your breath.

Single Whip

Step up to the Seven Stars

Here, you rise up from Descending Single Whip and step forward, bringing the two hands together as fists. In the final pose, your body shape is said to look like the seven stars that make up the Big Dipper constellation—the right leg is the tail that drops downward with your arms forming the rounded shape above.

1 Come up from Descending Single Whip, shifting more of your weight onto the left leg as you do so. Lift the right toes and turn the foot through a 90° angle to the left. Slide the foot closer to your left one, leaving about one and a half times your shoulder-width between them. Raise the left arm, dropping the elbow. Bring the hand into a loose tai chi fist. The right arm continues to extend, hand still in its beak shape.

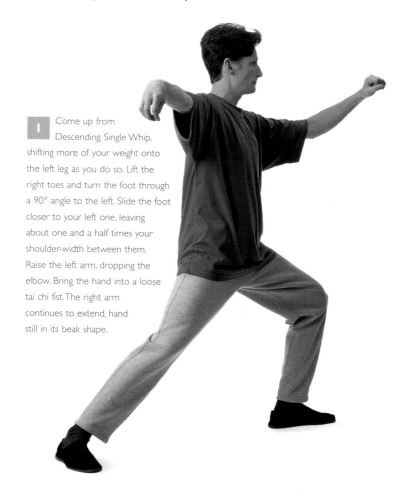

2 Move most of your weight onto the left leg. Let the right heel rise in preparation for the step. Lower the right arm, releasing the hand from the beak-shape. Move it forward, fingers pointing down. Start to bend the left elbow to bring the forearm closer to your body.

3 Step forward with the right foot, placing the heel down first. The foot should be at a 45° angle to the left one. At the same time, bring both forearms toward you, bending the elbows. As you bring the right arm in, make a fist with the right hand. Rest the right wrist on the left one, so that the hands are level with your shoulders and the thumb-side of both fists are pointing toward you. Keep 90 percent of your weight in the left leg. This is the cat stance.

Descending Single Whip

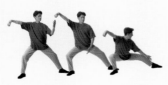

Step Back to Ride the Tiger

In this sequence, you step the right foot backward which requires good balance and a stable posture. Make sure that you place the toes down first, and then roll the rest of the foot onto the floor.

1 Keeping your weight on the left leg, turn the waist to the right and step back with the right foot. Place it at an angle of about 45° to the left one. At the same time, release your hands from the fists. Open out the arms and lower them to bring the hands level with the thighs, palms pointing backward.

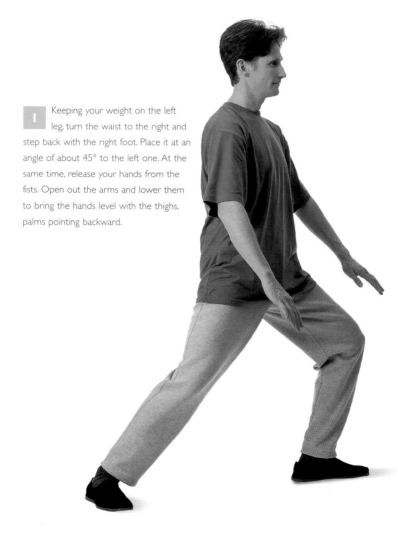

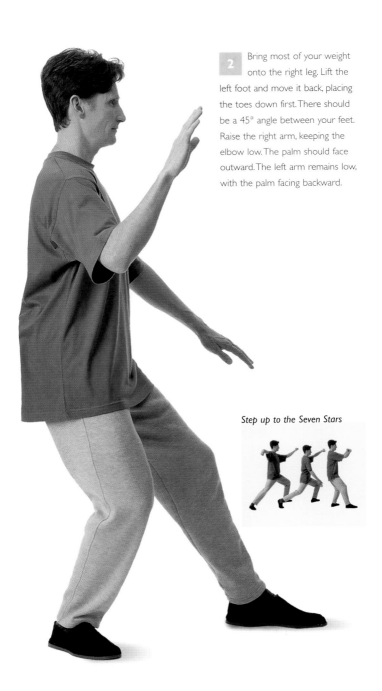

2 Bring most of your weight onto the right leg. Lift the left foot and move it back, placing the toes down first. There should be a 45° angle between your feet. Raise the right arm, keeping the elbow low. The palm should face outward. The left arm remains low, with the palm facing backward.

Step up to the Seven Stars

Turn and Sweep Lotus

This lengthy sequence involves turning the body through a full circle. Keep dropping your weight downward so that you maintain a stable posture. At the same time, make sure that your body remains relaxed and soft, particularly in the hips.

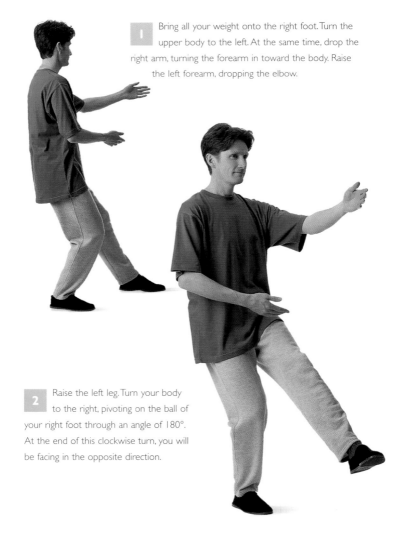

1 Bring all your weight onto the right foot. Turn the upper body to the left. At the same time, drop the right arm, turning the forearm in toward the body. Raise the left forearm, dropping the elbow.

2 Raise the left leg. Turn your body to the right, pivoting on the ball of your right foot through an angle of 180°. At the end of this clockwise turn, you will be facing in the opposite direction.

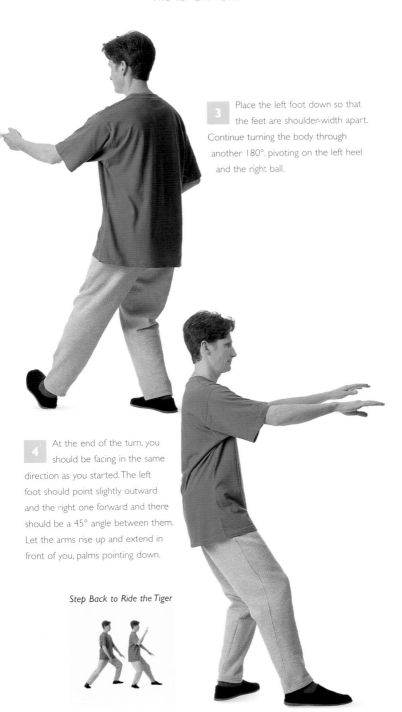

3 Place the left foot down so that the feet are shoulder-width apart. Continue turning the body through another 180°, pivoting on the left heel and the right ball.

4 At the end of the turn, you should be facing in the same direction as you started. The left foot should point slightly outward and the right one forward and there should be a 45° angle between them. Let the arms rise up and extend in front of you, palms pointing down.

Step Back to Ride the Tiger

Turn and Sweep Lotus

Here, you raise the right leg into a heel kick. Keep your movements slow and controlled at all times. Do not raise the leg high if you have problems with your lower back or find it hard to keep your balance.

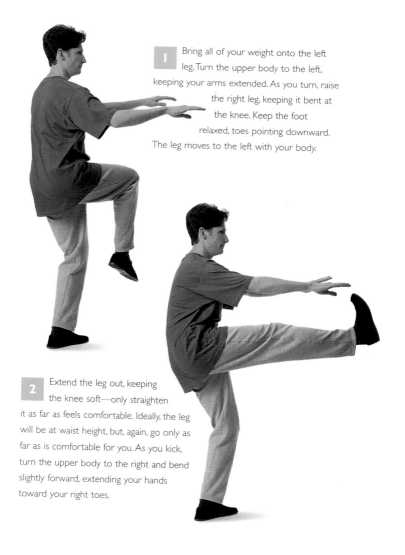

1 Bring all of your weight onto the left leg. Turn the upper body to the left, keeping your arms extended. As you turn, raise the right leg, keeping it bent at the knee. Keep the foot relaxed, toes pointing downward. The leg moves to the left with your body.

2 Extend the leg out, keeping the knee soft—only straighten it as far as feels comfortable. Ideally, the leg will be at waist height, but, again, go only as far as is comfortable for you. As you kick, turn the upper body to the right and bend slightly forward, extending your hands toward your right toes.

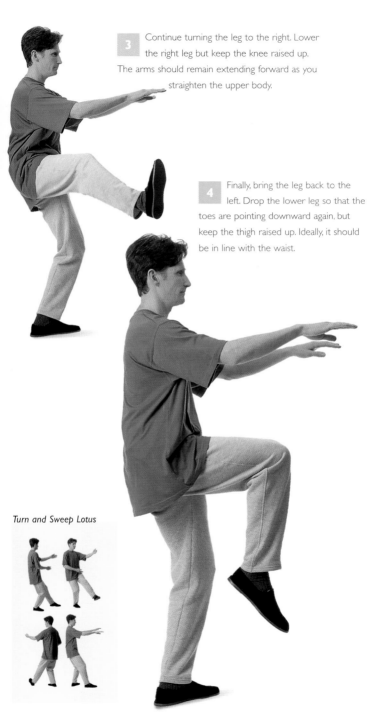

3 Continue turning the leg to the right. Lower the right leg but keep the knee raised up. The arms should remain extending forward as you straighten the upper body.

4 Finally, bring the leg back to the left. Drop the lower leg so that the toes are pointing downward again, but keep the thigh raised up. Ideally, it should be in line with the waist.

Turn and Sweep Lotus

Draw a Bow to Shoot the Tiger

This is a strong sequence that helps to ground you after the high kick. Keep the upper body relaxed. It will be easier to get the hands into alignment if you imagine you are holding a long staff.

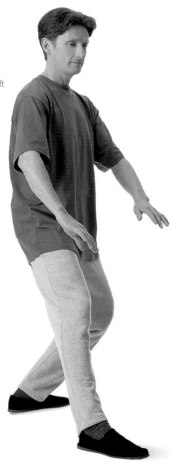

1 Keeping your weight in the left leg, move the right foot out and forward. Do not lean forward as you step. The right foot should be at right angles to the left one. Lower the arms, keeping the palms facing down. At the same time, turn the upper body to the right. About 90 percent of your weight should be on the left leg,.

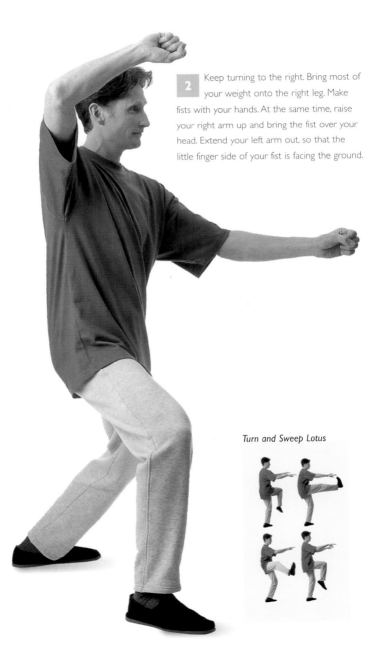

2 Keep turning to the right. Bring most of your weight onto the right leg. Make fists with your hands. At the same time, raise your right arm up and bring the fist over your head. Extend your left arm out, so that the little finger side of your fist is facing the ground.

Turn and Sweep Lotus

Step Forward, Deflect, Parry and Punch

This is the second time this sequence appears. The initial steps are different because you start with the right leg forward instead of the left one. The sequence leads into the closing movements of the form.

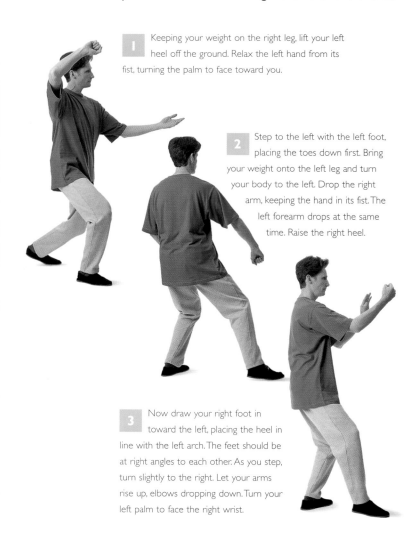

1 Keeping your weight on the right leg, lift your left heel off the ground. Relax the left hand from its fist, turning the palm to face toward you.

2 Step to the left with the left foot, placing the toes down first. Bring your weight onto the left leg and turn your body to the left. Drop the right arm, keeping the hand in its fist. The left forearm drops at the same time. Raise the right heel.

3 Now draw your right foot in toward the left, placing the heel in line with the left arch. The feet should be at right angles to each other. As you step, turn slightly to the right. Let your arms rise up, elbows dropping down. Turn your left palm to face the right wrist.

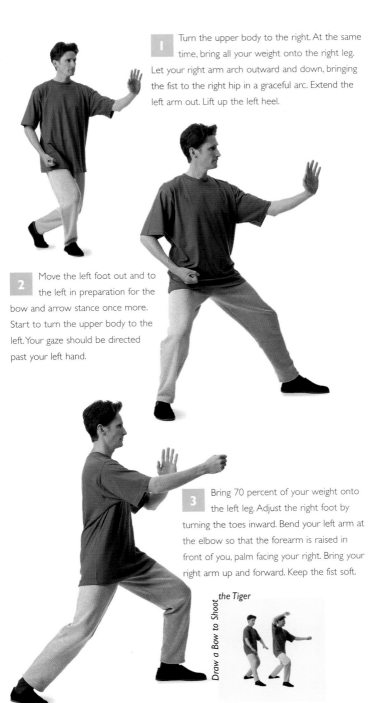

1 Turn the upper body to the right. At the same time, bring all your weight onto the right leg. Let your right arm arch outward and down, bringing the fist to the right hip in a graceful arc. Extend the left arm out. Lift up the left heel.

2 Move the left foot out and to the left in preparation for the bow and arrow stance once more. Start to turn the upper body to the left. Your gaze should be directed past your left hand.

3 Bring 70 percent of your weight onto the left leg. Adjust the right foot by turning the toes inward. Bend your left arm at the elbow so that the forearm is raised in front of you, palm facing your right. Bring your right arm up and forward. Keep the fist soft.

Draw a Bow to Shoot the Tiger

Withdraw and Push

The Punch sequence leads into Withdraw and Push. You release the hands from their fists, draw them into the body, and push out, in one rhythmic flow. The arm movement helps to loosen the wrists and elbows. Keep the shoulders relaxed as you push outward.

1 Turn the upper body to the left. Lower the left arm to bring the hand close to the right elbow, turning the palm upward. At the same time, raise the right forearm and release the right fist. Rotate the wrist to turn the right palm upward.

2 Increase the weight on the right leg to about 70 percent. Turn the upper body to the right. Draw back the right arm so the forearm passes over the left palm, but without touching it. Lower the left arm so both elbows are in front of you, palms up.

3 Turn the palms to face forward, keeping the wrists relaxed. Shift your weight until about 70 percent is on the left leg. Move the upper body forward, keeping the spine and head erect.

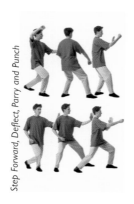

Step Forward, Deflect, Parry and Punch

Crossing Hands

This sequence draws energy into the body from the atmosphere. You move the feet back into the parallel stance, and you end the tai chi form in exactly the same place from which you started. End with 60 percent of your weight on the left leg, 40 percent of the right.

1 Bring most of your weight onto the right leg. Relax the wrists so that your hands are flat, palms facing downward. Keep the shoulders relaxed, and your spine upright.

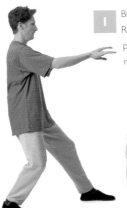

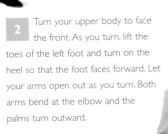

2 Turn your upper body to face the front. As you turn, lift the toes of the left foot and turn on the heel so that the foot faces forward. Let your arms open out as you turn. Both arms bend at the elbow and the palms turn outward.

Withdraw and Push

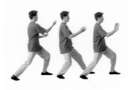

3 Move the right foot back, parallel with the left and a shoulder-width apart. Lower the hands, then raise them in a circular movement, crossing right wrist over left.

Completion

The final steps of the tai chi form are calming, but also strengthening. As you move into the final pose, check that your posture is balanced and stable. Make sure that your head and spine are in alignment, with the chin and tail bone tucked in. Your shoulders should be relaxed, arms held slightly away from the body. Your hips and knees should be soft, and the feet are flat on the floor. Spend a few moments enjoying standing in this way.

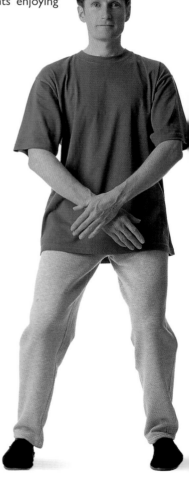

1 Lower the hands, reversing your hands so that the left now crosses over the right. Shift your weight so that it is equally distributed between the two feet.

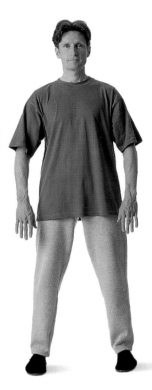

2 Uncross the hands and move them to your sides, palms facing backward. Keep a space between the arms and the sides of your body.

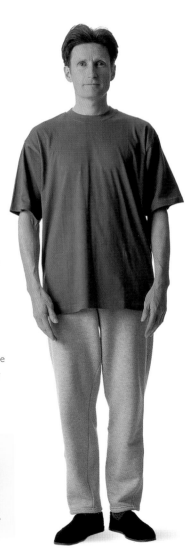

3 Bring more of your weight onto the left leg. Raise the right toes and draw in the heel. Then move your weight onto the right leg and do the same with your left foot. Your heels should be close together, toes pointing outward. Bring your arms closer into the body. Shift your weight until it is equally balanced. This is the end of the form.

Crossing Hands

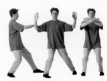

A Deeper Practice

At the end of a tai chi session you should feel grounded and relaxed, refreshed in body and soul. In this state, you are better equipped to deal with the stresses and vicissitudes of daily life. But it is best not to rush straight from your tai chi practice back into the frenetic round of work and home. Take time to enjoy the sense of well-being and harmony that tai chi brings.

If possible, find yourself a good tai chi teacher. You may have to try several classes to find one that suits you. Some masters of the form emphasize its health-giving qualities; others stress its applications as a martial art. Most good teachers will have an interest in these dual aspects, and each approach can give you greater understanding.

Going to a class will give you a chance to do partner work. This, too, is a means of deepening your practice. The discipline of working with another practitioner can open up new vistas to you.

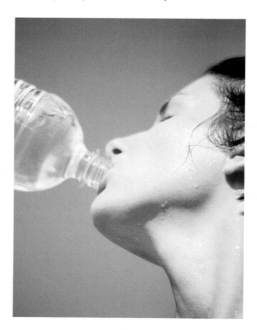

■ It is a good idea to have a drink of fruit juice, herbal tea, or water after doing tai chi or any form of exercise. Keeping well-hydrated is essential to health.

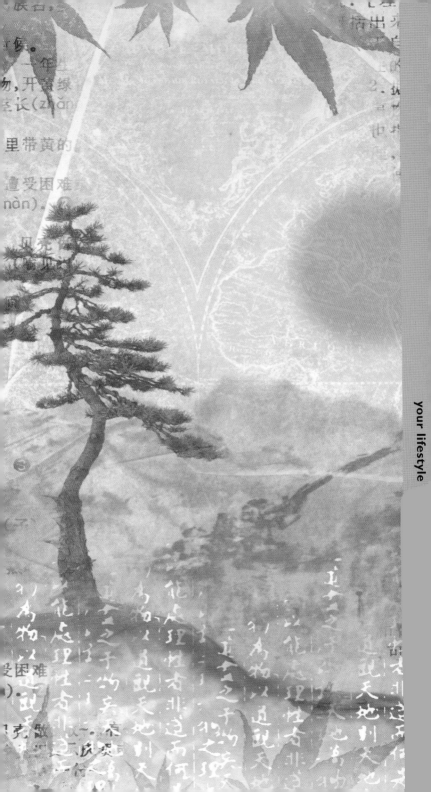

your lifestyle

Tai Chi and Your Lifestyle

Your tai chi practice does not finish when you reach the end of the form. The benefits and the lessons of your tai chi practice should, in time, seep into your daily life, like water into a sponge. You might, for example, find yourself drawing on the tai chi virtues of patience, precision, and thoughtful awareness to solve problems and deal with difficult situations. You can then reinvest these abilities in your practice: work on your tai chi, and your tai chi will work on you.

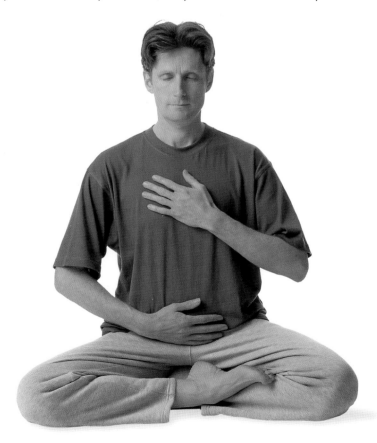

Using Tai Chi Principles

Tai chi is a not an end in itself. The point of tai chi, the reason for doing it, is to improve the quality of your life in all its aspects. Tai chi can help you to think more deeply, act more creatively, work more efficiently, relax more effectively, and live more fully.

The physical benefits alone are worth the investment. Most of us, for example, are unaware of the damage we do to ourselves simply by standing very badly. The most rudimentary grasp of tai chi posture would help protect against the chronic back pain which is endemic in the West. The same is true of tai chi breathing. Our breath is a unique body process: it is something that happens automatically, but which we control by the mind. There can be no doubt that we would be healthier if we only trained ourselves to breathe better at all times.

You can practice tai chi standing or breathing at any moment of the day—on a bus, in a store, sitting at a computer screen. The same applies to tai chi movement. An ordinary day is filled with repetitive activities that can be done better or made easier by applying the principles of tai chi. You will not find "tai chi ironing" in any of the classic texts, but it is a perfectly proper application of the form: stand in relaxed tai chi posture; then, as you bring the iron back and forth, let the movement unfold from your center and synchronize it with the turning of your waist. You could apply tai chi movement to sweeping a floor, digging the garden, painting a wall...

The same applies to mental activities. The concentration, that a practitioner brings to the form—as well as the element of self-monitoring and the attention to detail—these are intellectual virtues with broad applications. It is no exaggeration to say that tai chi can add some new dimension or other to all useful forms of human activity.

■ *The focus, balance, and breathing skills that you develop in tai chi can enhance any sporting activity, from walking in the park to scaling a rock face.*

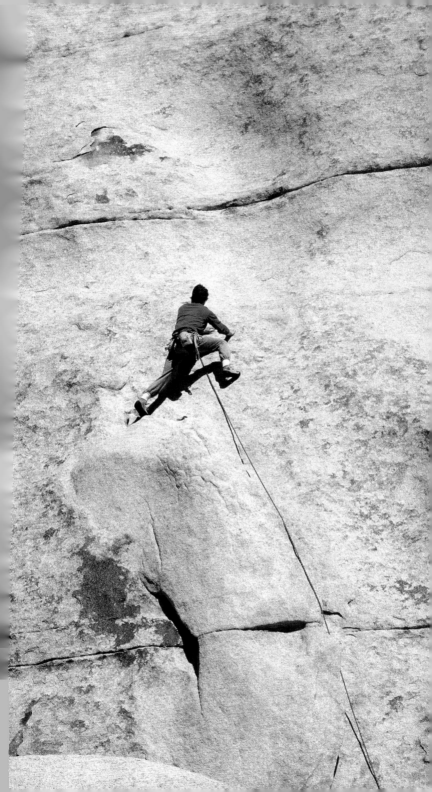

A Healing Pause

Most people don't get enough rest. If you continue to be active when you are tired, then you deplete your energy reserves and disturb the body's capacity to heal itself.

These exercises are quick and easy ways to replenish your reserves, and they can be done at any point during the day. They take just a few minutes, but can really help if you are feeling low, tired, or under pressure. If you are somewhere public, then simply drop your shoulders, sit or stand upright, and take some deep breaths. Breathing is the best way to improve your well-being in an instant.

LETTING GO

Lie down, keeping your body in a straight line. Place a cushion under your knees to relieve any pressure on the back. Rest the hands comfortably on the chest and upper abdomen. Now let your weight sink down—let the ground support you as you release tension from your muscles. As you relax, gradually deepen your breathing. As you breathe in, feel your hands rise. As the hands fall, imagine you are sinking deeper into the ground. Do this for two or three minutes, then get up slowly.

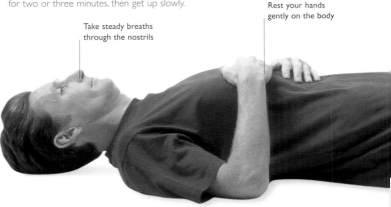

Rest your hands gently on the body

Take steady breaths through the nostrils

A QUIET MOMENT

This meditation focuses your attention on the lower and middle tan tiens. Simply concentrating on these areas helps to direct chi into them. The exercise also requires you to sit in silence—itself a healing thing to do. This is a lovely way to end a tai chi practice. You can also use it any time you need to bring stillness into your day.

1 Sit comfortably on the floor or in a chair. Rest one hand on top of the other just below your navel. Close your eyes and bring your attention to the area under your hands. Simply notice any sensations you experience here as you breathe. Do this for a minute or two.

2 Leave the right hand on the lower abdomen, rest the left one in the middle of the chest. As you breathe, see if you can bring your attention to both areas. If this feels tricky, focus on either area or let your attention move between them. Again, try to be aware of the sensations without trying to change them.

Focus the mind

The fingers are not touching

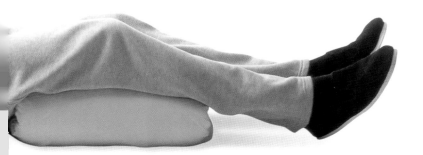

Simple De-Stresser

When we are stressed, we lose our sense of groundedness. Stress equals upward movement: our shoulders hunch up, our voices become loud and shrill, panic rises from the stomach to the chest to the throat. This exercise, which is taken from chi kung, helps to bring energy back down the body. It reestablishes your connection with the earth and helps to restore your sense of calm.

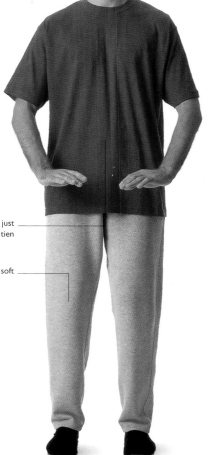

I Stand with your feet hip-width apart and firmly planted on the floor. Shift your weight until it is distributed equally between the feet. Bring the hands to just below the lower tan tien, fingers relaxed and palms pointing down to the ground.

Hands are held just below the tan tien

Keep the knees soft

WATCH THE SHOULDERS

Relax your shoulders before you start, drawing the blades down the back and slightly inward. Do not let them tense or rise up with the arms; keep them relaxed and let your arms float upward.

2 Bend your elbows and slowly move the hands up the center of the body before opening them out to the sides. As you bring the hands up, imagine you are drawing energy from the earth and directing it through the body. At the same time, bend your knees.

3 Bring the forearms into the center of the body, then lower them to just below the tan tien again. Imagine you are drawing the energy back down the body and returning it to the earth. Straighten your legs, but keep the knees soft. Repeat the actions for a couple of minutes, coordinating the arms and legs in a smooth rhythm. Return your hands to your sides and breathe.

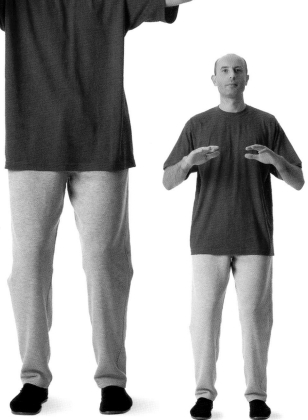

Quick Releasers for Tired Legs

Standing still for long periods is not good for you. Your circulation slows down and this can make your legs feel tired and aching. If you are on your feet for long periods, try walking on the spot from time to time. At the end of a long day, do these exercises to enliven the legs and mobilize the joints. You could also give yourself a quick foot rub to get energy flowing back to this often-neglected area of the body.

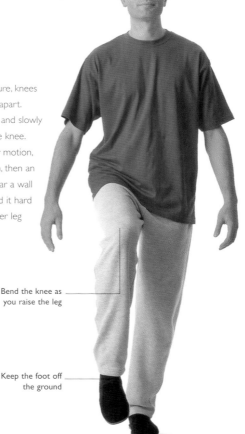

RAISE THE KNEE

Stand in a relaxed, upright posture, knees slightly bent and feet hip-width apart. Bring your weight onto one leg and slowly raise the other one, bending the knee. Move the entire leg in a circular motion, working in a clockwise direction, then an counterclockwise one. Stand near a wall and use it for support if you find it hard to balance. Repeat with the other leg

Bend the knee as you raise the leg

Keep the foot off the ground

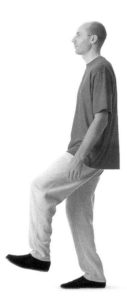

KICKING OUT

This is a good way of exercising the feet and ankles, and it can also help to release pent-up energy or emotion from the body.

1 Lift your leg and bend the knee. Extend the lower leg forward, pointing the toe in a relaxed kick. Swing the leg backward and forward a few times—do not lock the knee.

2 Now turn the toes to point upward. Again, swing the leg backward and forward a few times, leading with the heel. Do not make any abrupt movements. Repeat Steps 1 and 2 on the other leg.

ROTATING ANKLES

Lift your leg again and extend it forward. Make circles with your feet, rotating the ankles. Work gently in a clockwise direction three times, then repeat in an clockclockwise direction. Do the same on the other leg.

Do not lock the knee at any point

Keep the foot flat as you circle it

In the Office

Working in an office can be bad for your health, especially if you sit at a computer. Office workers tend to remain in the same position for long periods, which can make the circulation sluggish. Get into the habit of checking your posture, and shift if you are uncomfortable. Get up and walk around every hour or so, and make sure that every day you find some time and a space to stretch out once a day.

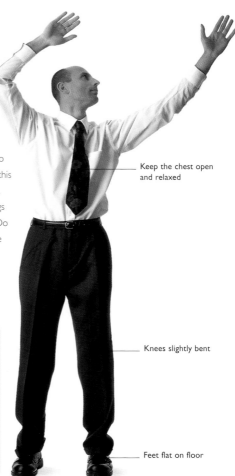

ARM CIRCLES

Stand erect, feet hip-width apart and arms by your sides. Sweep your hands to one side and then up over your head and down again, in a large circular motion. Work gently, and do not wrench or twist the body. Do this a couple of times in each direction. Repeat and this time bend your legs into a squat as your arms rise up. Do this twice in each direction. Breathe deeply as you exercise.

Keep the chest open and relaxed

Knees slightly bent

Feet flat on floor

FOOT WORK

While sitting at your desk, take off your shoes and place the feet flat on the floor. Lift the heels up and hold for a moment, then return them to the floor and lift the balls and toes up. Do this five or six times, several times a day.

ARM SWINGS

Now turn your waist to one side letting your arms follow the movement—tai-chi style—as you do so. Turn back to the front and then turn to the other side, again letting the arms follow. Do this for 30 seconds to one minute, breathing deeply. Work gently, and do not force the movement farther than feels natural. Keep the knees slightly bent all the time.

FORWARD BEND

From a standing position, bend forward very slowly. Let your arms hang down. Keep the legs upright, knees slightly bent. Try to fold forward from the hips, letting the bend move slowly up the spine. Do not go any farther than is comfortable. To come up, bend your knees and slowly uncurl your spine from the base to the top. Lift your head up last.

Head drops down

Arms held out to the sides

SHAKE-OUT

Try the shake-out exercise to release tension and frustration. Stand in a relaxed tai chi posture. Bring your arms away from your body and gently shake them for a few moments. Bring all your weight onto one leg. Lift the other off the floor and shake it out. Then repeat with the other leg. Rest in the standing position for a few minutes.

In the Car

Sitting in the same position in cramped conditions can cause tension in the mind as well as the body. When driving, see every traffic signal and every gridlock as a chance to relax. Whenever you have a stationary moment or two, place your feet flat on the floor, relax your shoulders, and lean back into the seat. Now take three deep breaths. If you are on a long journey, stop every couple of hours to stretch out.

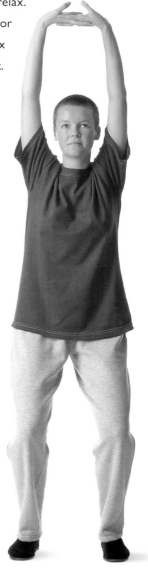

FULL-BODY STRETCH

Stand in a relaxed upright posture, with your feet hip-width apart and knees soft. Raise your arms above your head, interlock your fingers and turn the palms to face upward. Keep the shoulders relaxed. Now, bend the knees to lower yourself into a squat as you continue to stretch upward with the arms. Take a deep breath in, and exhale strongly. Then straighten the legs, unlock the fingers, and lower the arms to your side. Repeat two or three times more.

CLAPPING

This is a good exercise for releasing
tension in the shoulders and opening the
chest, so that you can breathe freely.

1 Stand in a relaxed way, with your
arms hanging down by your sides.
Move the arms back and clap your hands
behind your back.

2 Now bring the arms forward and
up, until they are level with your
shoulders. Clap the hands. Repeat Steps 1
and 2 a few times.

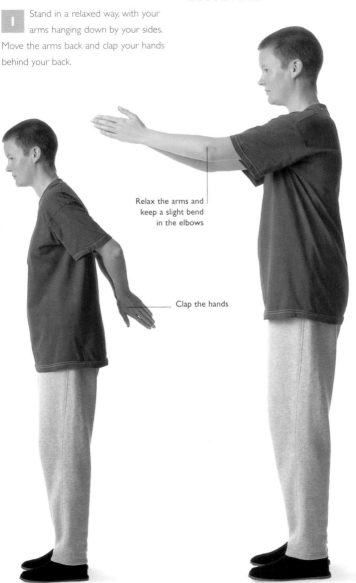

Relax the arms and
keep a slight bend
in the elbows

Clap the hands

Glossary

acupuncture Chinese therapy that involves inserting fine needles into points on the body's energy channels to promote the flow of chi.

application Tai chi developed as a "soft" martial art in which energy is directed inward. However, the actions can be speeded up and adapted for self-defense. Some of these martial-art applications are evident from the name given to the sequence—for example, Right toe kick or Push. Others are less obvious—the upper arm in Diagonal Flying, for example, can be used to strike the throat of an opponent coming from behind.

chang san feng The 13th-century Taoist sage who is credited as being the founder of tai chi. His original style was known as Wu Dang Mountain Tai Chi or The Twelve Chi Disruption Forms.

Cheng Man-ching Cheng Man-ching was an innovative 20th-century teacher who helped to popularize tai chi in both China and the West. He modified the traditional Yang style of tai chi, developing the short form that is practiced all over the world today.

chi The vital energy that gives us life, strength and health according to Chinese philosophy. This animating force flows through all things in the universe. Tai chi is practiced to help chi to flow freely through meridians in the body, which promotes good health. Chi is sometimes written as qi.

Dr Chi Chiang-tao Dr Chi Chiang-tao studied tai chi with Cheng Man-ching and became a respected teacher himself. He created a variation to his master's short form, adding several new sequences from the Yang long form. He believed that this change made the form more beneficial for health. His variation is widely practiced.

chi kung An energy practice that is related to tai chi, and predates it by several centuries. Chi kung exercises are performed standing up, and usually involve a minimum of movement. Like tai chi, they seek to improve the flow of chi through the body. Chi kung is sometimes written as Qigong.

chinese medicine Traditional Chinese Medicine (TCM) is a complete health system that encompasses acupuncture, Chinese herbalism, and exercises such as tai chi and chi kung. The flow of chi is seen as essential to good health by all branches of TCM.

form Tai chi exercises are performed in a strictly choreographed order. This is known as a form. The form varies depending on the style of tai chi.

master The term master is used to mean someone who is not only physically adept at a practice but who has fully understood and embraced all its many aspects.

meridians Invisible channels in the body through which chi passes. There are 12 main meridians in acupuncture, most of which are named after the vital organs to which they are connected. They include the heart meridian, kidney meridian, and liver meridian.

pushing hands Tai chi sparring exercises that are done with a partner. In a pushing hands exercise, you yield in order to neutralize an incoming push and then move forward into a push yourself. Many tai chi classes include pushing hands work, which can help to develop sensitivity. Pushing hands is also practiced as a gentle sport, in which the aim is to upset your opponent's balance. It can be studied to competition level.

rooting This term means being creating a strong connection with the ground. When your feet are firmly planted on the floor, they provide a strong base and give your posture stability, which is an essential part of tai chi.

softening Tai chi teachers use this term frequently. When you soften an area of the body, you relax it both physically and mentally. All the joints in tai chi should be soft.

style There are different types of tai chi. This book concentrates on Yang-style short form, which is the most widely practiced style of tai chi. You can also learn Yang long form, as well as Chen style, Wu style, Wu Shi style, Sun style and Beijing style.

sword form Tai chi can be practiced with a sword. This can help to improve your ability to move the body as a single unit. But you need to have a good grounding of tai chi before you learn sword form.

tai chi chuan The full name for tai chi. Tai means "great," chi means "life force" and chuan means "fist." Together the words can be loosely translated as "great ultimate power" or perhaps "great strength of opposites." Tai chi chuan is sometimes written as Taijiquan.

tan tien This refers to the lower tan tien, the area in the body where your chi is stored. It lies just beneath the navel and about an inch in toward the spine. In tai chi, all your movements should be guided by the lower tan tien. There are two other tan tiens in the body. The middle tan tien is your heart area, which is just behind the solar plexus. The upper tan tien is situated in the forehead, between the eyebrows. It is often known as the third eye.

taoism Chinese philosophy which is a way of understanding the way the universe works. Taoists believe that the world is in a constant state of flux—the Tao or Way. Only by yielding to the Tao can one find happiness. The concepts of yin and yang are central to Taoist belief.

yin and yang The opposing energetic forces that make up the universe. Yin is the energy of the earth. It is feminine, dark, receptive energy which is concerned with stability and structure. Yang is the energy of the sky, or heavens. It is seen as masculine, light, creative energy which is concerned with movement and change.

yung chuan The yung chuan is a point in the center in the ball of the foot. Chi travels through this point into the earth. Tai chi teachers say that you should concentrate your weight here.

Useful Addresses

USA

Tai Chi Foundation
657a Main Street
Laurel MD 20707
Tel: 212 645 7010
www.taichifoundation.org

USA National Tai Chi Chuan Federation
806-808 Main Street
Manchester CT 06040
Tel: 860 646 6818
www.usataichi.org

CANADA

The Canadian Taijiquan Federation
PO Box 421
Milton
Ontario L9T 4Z1
www.canadiantaijiquanfederation.ca

EUROPE

Tai Chi Union for Great Britain *and*
Taijiquan and Qigong Federation for Europe
1 Littlemill Drive
Balmoral Gardens
Crookston
Glasgow G53 7GF
Tel: +44 (0) 141 810 3482
www.taijiquan-qigong.com

Fédération Française des Tai Chi Chuan
78 rue Saint Honoré,
75001 Paris.
Tel: +33 (0)1 45 43 03 96

Stichting Taijiquan Nederland
Postbus 13 26 4
3507 LG
Utrecht
Netherlands
Tel: +31 (0)30 289 6336
www.taijiquan.nl

AUSTRALIA

Tai Chi Association of Australia
PO Box 9
Morwell
Victoria 3840
www.taichiaustralia.com

INTERNATIONAL

International Yang Style Tai Chi Chuan Association
4076, 148th Avenue NE
Redmond
WA 98052
Tel: 425 869 1185
www.yangfamilytaichi.com

Taiji Club
PO Box 564
Douglassville
PA 19518
Tel: 610 689 0571
http://taijiquanclub.com

WEBSITES

Many tai teachers now have their own websites, giving details of the practice and the particular style that they teach. The following websites contain lists of teachers, and can be a good way of finding a class in your area:

Taiji Germany
www.taiji.de

Tai Chi Network
www.taichinetwork.org

Tai Chi Finder UK
www.taichifinder.co.uk

Further Reading

TAI CHI

Cheng Man-ching. **Cheng Tzu's Thirteen Treatises on Tai Chi Chuan,** translated by Ben Lo and Martin Inn, North Atlantic Books, 1993

Chuen, Master Lam Kam. **Step-by-Step Tai Chi** Gaia Books, 1994

Clark, Angus. **The Complete Illustrated Guide to Tai Chi,** Element, 2000

Crompton, Paul. **The Elements of Tai Chi,** Element Books, 1990

Docherty, Dan. **Complete T'ai Chi Ch'uan,** Crowood Press, 1997

Kauz, Herman. **Push Hands: The Handbook for Noncompetitive Tai Chi Practice with a Partner** Overlook Press, 2001

Kiew Kit, Wong. **The Complete Book of Tai Chi Ch'uan,** Element Books, 1996

Lam, Paul and Horstman, Judith. **Overcoming Arthritis: How to Relieve Pain and Restore Mobility through a Unique Tai Chi Programme** DK Publishing, 2002

Lowenthal, Wolfe. **There Are No Secrets: Professor Cheng Man-Ching and HIs Tai Chi Chuan** North Atlantic Books, 1991

Peck, Alan. **T'ai Chi: The Essential Introductory Guide,** Vermilion, 1999

CHI KUNG

Clark, Angus. **Secrets of QiGong,** DK 2001

Dong, Paul. **Chi Gong,** Paragon House, 1990

Frantzis, Bruce Kumar. **Opening the Energy Gates of Your Body,** North Atlantic Books, 1997

Kit, Wong Kiew. **Chi Kung for Health & Vitality,** Element, 1997

McRitchie, J. **The Art of Chi Kung,** Element, 1993

Reid, Daniel. **Harnessing the Power of the Universe, A Comprehensive Guide to the Principles and Practice of Qigong,** Simon & Schuster, 1998

Wang, Simon, and Liu, Julius L. **Qi Gong for Health & Longevity** The East Health Development Group, 1995

MARTIAL ARTS

Finn, Michael. **Martial Arts: A Complete Illustrated History,** Stanley Paul, 1988

Reid, Howard, and Croucher, Michael. **The Way of the Warrior** Century Publishing, 1983

CHINESE PHILOSOPHY

Fung Yu-lan. **A Short History of Chinese Philosophy,** The Free Press, 1995

Lao Tzu. **Tao Te Ching,** translated by D.C. Lau, Penguin Classics, 1985

JOURNALS

Qi Journal—The Journal of Traditional Eastern Health and Fitness
Graphics Inc, Box 18476, Anaheim Hills
CA 92817
Tel: 714 779 1796
www.qi-journal.com

Taijiquan Journal
PO Box 80538
Minneapolis
MN 55408, USA
Tel: 612 822 5760
www.taijiquanjournal.com

T'ai Chi Magazine
Wayfarer Publications
2601 Silver Ridge Avenue
Los Angeles
CA 90039
Tel: 800 888 9119
www.tai-chi.com

Qi Magazine
Tse Qigong Centre
PO Box 59
Altrincham
WA15 8FS, UK
Tel: +44 (0) 161 929 4485
www.qimagazine.com

Index

ACKNOWLEDGMENTS

With thanks to Jonathan Bastable, for his help in producing this book
And also with gratitude to all the tai chi practitioners who appear i
the photographs.